Sylvie McCracken of HollywoodHomestead.com
Copyright 2014 Sylvie McCracken

DISCLAIMER AND COPYRIGHT INFORMATION

This book is not to be considered a replacement for medical advice, diagnosis, or treatment. Please always use your best judgment and seek the advice of your health professionals as needed.

By reading this guide, you agree that neither the author nor the author's company is responsible for your results relating to any information presented in the guide. Furthermore, any statements or claims about the possible health benefits conferred by any foods or supplements have not been evaluated by the US Food and Drug Administration and are therefore not intended to diagnose, treat, cure, or prevent any disease.

Most of the outbound links here and on my websites are purely for informational purposes. However, I do earn a small commission on some of the links to books and products referenced here and on my website. As always, I will never recommend a resource I cannot personally vouch for.

No part of this publication shall be reproduced, transmitted, or sold in whole or in part in any form, without the prior written consent from the author, Sylvie McCracken.

This eBook is licensed for your personal enjoyment only. It may not be resold or given away. If you would like to share this book with another person, please purchase an additional copy for each recipient. Thank you for respecting the hard work of the author.

Copyright Hollywood Homestead. All rights reserved.

Contents

9 ABOUT THE AUTHOR

10 REAL FOOD SUCCESS STORIES
- Sylvie's Journey ⋯ 10
- Eric's Journey ⋯ 14

15 INTRODUCTION
- What is Gelatin? ⋯ 16
- Glycine and Proline: The Basic Components of Collagen ⋯ 16
- How Is Gelatin Made? ⋯ 19
- Bone Broth as a Source of Gelatin ⋯ 20
- Why Eat Gelatin? ⋯ 24
- How to Choose Gelatin ⋯ 26
- How Gelatin Nourishes Each Part of Your Body ⋯ 28

31 GELATIN FOR BONE HEALTH
- What Are Bones? ⋯ 32
- Common Bone Problems and Diseases ⋯ 33
- The Importance of Collagen for Bone Health ⋯ 36
- Gelatin for Healing Bones ⋯ 36

39 GELATIN FOR JOINT HEALTH
- What Are Our Joints Made Of? ⋯ 39
- The Proof is in the (Gelatin) Pudding ⋯ 40
- Gelatin + Vitamin C for Healthy Joints ⋯ 41

43 GELATIN FOR GUT HEALTH
- What is Leaky Gut Syndrome? ⋯ 43
- What Makes a Gut Become Leaky? ⋯ 44
- Why You Should Be Worried About Leaky Gut ⋯ 46
- Signs You Have a Leaky Gut ⋯ 47
- How to Diagnose Food Sensitivities and Leaky Gut Syndrome ⋯ 48
- How to Repair Leaky Gut ⋯ 51
- So, What Does Gelatin Have to do with Repairing Leaky Gut? ⋯ 53

54 GELATIN FOR WEIGHT LOSS

- Gelatin Regulates Blood Sugar Levels — 54
- Gelatin Inhibits Sugar Cravings — 57
- Gelatin Reduces Appetite — 57
- Gelatin Boosts Muscle Formation — 58

59 GELATIN FOR THE BRAIN

- Gelatin Calms the Body — 59
- Gelatin for Balancing Cortisol Levels — 60
- Gelatin and Mood — 62

63 GELATIN FOR SKIN HEALTH AND BEAUTY

- Gelatin for Skin Health — 64
- Gelatin for Wrinkles — 66
- Gelatin for Cellulite — 68
- Gelatin for Hair — 69
- Gelatin for Nails — 71
- Super Simple Skin Care Routine — 73

74 GELATIN FOR DENTAL HEALTH

- Anatomy of the Teeth — 74
- Why Brushing Won't Stop Tooth Decay — 76
- Weston A. Price Links Tooth Decay to Diet — 77
- How to Cure Tooth Decay with Diet — 78
- Squeezable Remineralizing Toothpaste Recipe — 79
- Tooth Healing Is Possible — 82

83 RECIPES

86 GUIDE TO MAKING GELATIN-RICH BONE BROTH

- Making Sense of Bone Quality — 87
- Different Types of Bone Broth: — 89
- Different Methods of Cooking Bone Broth: — 90
- How to Store Bone Broth — 94
- Troubleshooting: Why didn't my broth gel? — 94

97 SIDE DISH RECIPES

Pumpkin Purée 98
Braised Brussels Sprouts with Bacon 99
Sauteéd Chard 100
Glazed Carrots 101
Root Veggie Mash 102

103 SOUPS

Chicken Soup 104
Creamy Butternut Squash Soup 105
Sweet Potato Soup 106
Cream of Chicken Soup with lemongrass 107
"Tortilla" Soup 108

109 CONDIMENTS AND SAUCES

Ketchup 109
Mayonnaise 111
BBQ Sauce 112
Demi-Glace 113
Gravy 114

115 "JELLO" RECIPES

Orange Jello 116
Strawberry Jello 117
Blueberry Jello 118
Lemon Jello 119
Hibiscus Tea Jello 120
Kombucha Jello 121

122 GUMMIES

Strawberry Lemonade Gummies 123
Strawberry Cream Gummies 124
Lemon Gummies 125
Orange Gummy Bears 126
Blueberry Gummies 127
Tangerine Gummies 128

The Gelatin Secret

129 DAIRY FREE ICE CREAMS

- Mango Ice Cream — 130
- Lemon Ice Cream — 131
- Maple Banana Ice Cream — 133
- Strawberry Ice Cream — 134
- Vanilla Chocolate Chip Ice Cream — 135

136 DAIRY FREE SMOOTHIES

- Chocolate Banana Smoothie — 137
- Go Green Smoothie — 138
- Pumpkin Banana Smoothie — 139
- Pineapple Smoothie — 140
- Cucumber Avocado Smoothie — 141

142 DAIRY-FREE PUDDINGS AND CUSTARD

- Coconut Pudding — 143
- Pumpkin Pudding — 144
- Chocolate Pudding — 145
- Custard — 146
- Banana Cinnamon Pudding — 147
- Pumpkin Chocolate Mousse — 148
- Crème Brûlée — 149

150 MARSHMALLOWS

- Cinnamon Covered Marshmallows (with chocolate dipped option) — 150
- Chocolate Dip — 151

152 REFERENCES

SECTION 01 — HOLLYWOOD HOMESTEAD

About the Author

Sylvie was raised in Argentina but currently lives in Los Angeles where she juggles a fast-paced career as an Executive Assistant to an Oscar-winning actor while managing to get the real food word out to celebrities and civilians alike.

Sylvie and her husband Eric each lost over 60 lbs in the first year of adopting a real foods diet. You can read about their Real Food Success Stories.

On weekends, Sylvie, Eric, and their three kids can be found in the kitchen, the garden, the beach, or hiking, and sometimes a combo of all of the above. You can find out more about their lifestyle at the blog www.hollywoodhomestead.com and follow them on Facebook, Twitter, Pinterest, and Instagram. Sign up for our newletter at: www.hollywoodhomestead.com/sign-up

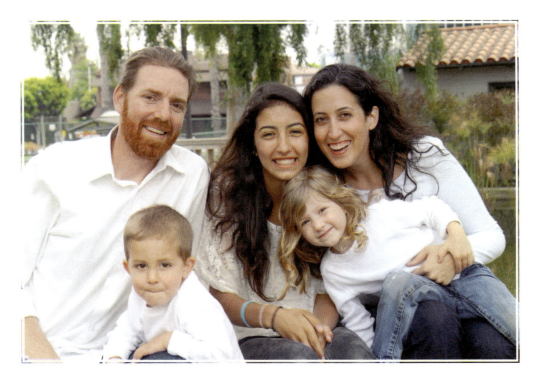

Real Food Success Stories

SYLVIE'S JOURNEY

I've lost 65 lbs with real food but, really, that's just the cherry on top.

I didn't get into the real food lifestyle to lose weight. I'd sort of given up on the weight-loss front. After hitting age 30 and having had 3 kids, I assumed there's only so much one can do.

I was not an overweight kid but I was definitely a health disaster. I ate a low-fat vegetarian diet for most of my childhood and consumed mostly soy and wheat with a few lentils thrown in for good measure. By age 15 my list of diagnoses was impressive and the medications were starting to pile up:

* Polycystic ovarian syndrome

* Chronic Amenhorrea = Rx: birth control

* Hypothyroid = Rx: Synthroid

* Tonsillitis and strep throat at least yearly = Rx: many rounds of Amoxicillin, later very high recurring doses of penicillin and finally a tonsillectomy

* Chronic allergic rhinitis = Rx: cortisone nasal spray and decongestants (which I became addicted to) and eventually nasal polyps which were surgically removed during my teen years in addition to cryosurgery on my adenoids. Fun times.

* Allergic to just about everything = Rx: allergy shots every 4 days starting as a pre-teen that I would self administer after school, and anaphylactic shock that landed me in the emergency room multiple times

* Epstein-Barr virus (aka "mono") multiple times = Rx: rest, hope and prayer (ha!)

* All of this was in addition to a heart condition I was born with

called supraventricular tachycardia for which I was on beta blockers and other random things that never worked until I had my heart catheter ablation when I was 21.

Comprehensive diagnosis: HOT MESS

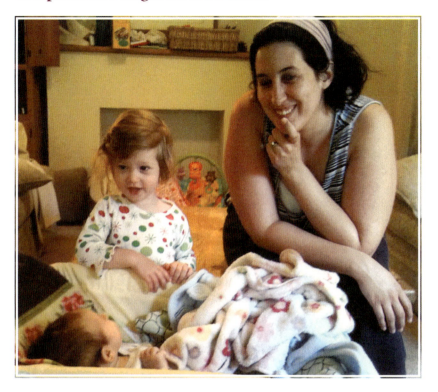

My medical file was a FAT one (pun intended)! Seriously, when my mom handed it off to me a few years ago, even I was shocked.

My experiment with the paleo diet came out of desperation since my thyroid symptoms (fatigue being the most crippling one) were persistent and severe despite my lab work being "normal". The first 30 days of the transition to paleo were *not* easy. My body was not used to so much animal protein and fat, and I was dealing with mad cravings for sugar and wheat. Finding the time, energy and money to do more shopping, cooking and dishes while juggling the usual madness of life definitely took some effort for both me and my husband Eric.

* We made mistakes.

* We got frustrated.

* But, we stuck with it.

I lost 65 lbs with paleo. The craziest part was that I wasn't focusing on weight loss at all.

I realize that there are many ways to lose weight. I've tried many of them myself: calorie counting, low fat, more exercise, low carb, Slim Fast, cortisol regulating supplements, among others. Some of them were seemingly successful, but I'd eventually gain the few pounds I lost right back.

You see, being overweight or underweight is often not the problem. It is a *symptom* of a problem. When you're body finds health, it will most likely self-adjust on the weight front quite a bit.

The improvements I found were well beyond weight loss:

- My cycle is like clockwork now. I'd asked countless MDs about this and only received shoulder shrugs and prescriptions for birth control. I was beginning to think regular cycles were a myth!

- My allergies are minimal and I no longer react to food after every single meal.

- My skin is clear.

- I no longer have yeast infections.

- My blood sugar (and hence mood) is finally regulated. I'm no longer "hangry" (hungry + angry) all the time!

- I sleep through the night and wake up with energy to work full time, take care of my family and run my blog and business.

- The bags under my eyes which I thought were hereditary and obsessively covered with makeup are gone (unless those little kids keep me up at night)

- My nails don't break as easily. My teeth are not translucent and I have not had a cavity since going paleo. This is someone that had a cavity at EVERY SINGLE dental visit—and no, my diet was not nothing but soda and pop tarts.

I was fat yet malnourished. It sounds paradoxical, but it's true.

My gut lining was so damaged that I was not absorbing many nutrients from food. Food really is medicine and, once I cleaned up my diet, I saw considerable improvements. Once I turned the dial up a notch and focused on healing my damaged gut, my health improved once again. This is because my body was finally able to make use of all that amazing, nutrient-dense food I was putting in my mouth.

HOLLYWOOD HOMESTEAD

I will always be a work in progress and have many years of damage to unravel. After three decades of consuming large amounts of soy, wheat and very little animal protein and fat, I can't just snap my fingers to regain my health — but I'm also not destined to be overweight and unhealthy for the rest of my life.

I encourage you to take your health in your hands, start reading labels of everything you consume, and focus on eating nutrient-dense foods and healing your body.

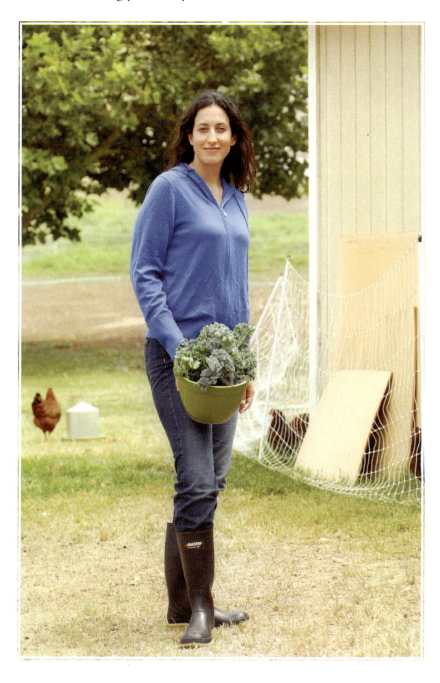

ERIC'S JOURNEY

Before we made the switch to real foods I felt slow and sluggish. I got winded easily. My joints hurt. The vision in my right eye was getting worse. I was on a hunger roller coaster — I went from too full to starving every few hours. It was tough to lose weight. My ideal weight in my mind was continuing to rise… 185… 195… I'll be happy under 200… 205 isn't that bad… everyone aspires to be at the weight they were when they got married, right? 205 is great! I feel fine.

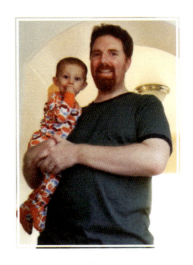

I was lying to myself. I was NOT feeling fine. I was tired. I had little energy.

I think the question is WHY? Why am I sluggish? Why do my joints hurt? Why is my vision getting worse? Why did I feel awful after eating and then starving a few hours later?

The standard answers to these questions are easy — you're getting old. You're overweight. That's just the way it is.

Standard answers didn't work for me: Reduce portion size. Exercise. Been there, done that. Lost weight and gained it right back again.

I wanted off the roller coaster.

I got off a plane from Abu Dhabi after 7 months of being without my wife and children. I weighed 235 pounds.

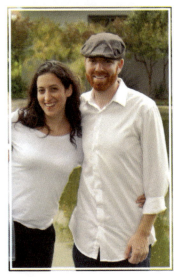

I didn't know it at the time, but we were about to find the answer. Both of us went about trying to get healthy. We started walking everywhere as much as we could. Eventually we stumbled upon paleo and found out about the gut connection. Sylvie started right away on paleo, but I was skeptical. Sylvie was starting to feel better so I decided to give it a try.

That was over 2 years ago. I am now 170 pounds. The vision in my right eye is fine. My joints don't hurt. I have energy again. I feel light on my feet. The best part? I am never hungry. I eat as much as I want and I don't think about calories. *I can't gain weight!* I got off the roller coaster and life is good. I see a field and I know I can sprint to the other side with my kids and actually beat them there. I have a 15 year old, so that's not easy! How many parents can say that? I feel like we stumbled upon a secret to good health that very few people believe or care to try.

The best way to start is to ask the right questions.

SECTION 02

HOLLYWOOD HOMESTEAD

Introduction

As a former lifelong vegetarian, one of the last things I thought I would do in my life is write an entire book on the topic of gelatin. If you told me before I started my real food journey that I'd be writing two eBooks and teaching online classes about nutrition and health, it would have cracked.me.up. I had no idea what I was doing. I didn't know where to start. I thought cayenne pepper and lemon would be the answer to all my problems.

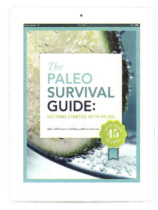

Over the last couple of years, I have studied, experimented, listened, written, argued, discussed, and absorbed as much information on nutrition and lifestyle as possible. I've swapped vacations for conferences and tv shows for seminars. I eat, sleep, and breathe paleo nutrition and lifestyle. I started my website and Facebook page because I just couldn't keep all of this to myself.

Every time my before and after photos are picked up in the interwebs, I have an influx of people coming to me saying *"you look great! I want to do this! How do I start?"* That is what led me to write my first ebook, *Paleo Made Easy: Getting your Family Started with the Optimal Healthy Lifestyle* (available at www.thepaleosurvivalguide.com)

In the last year or so, I've been sort of obsessed with micronutrients (vitamins and minerals) and nutrient density as well as gut health and absorption (since we aren't really what we eat but rather *what we absorb from what we eat*). This led me to research and play around with gelatin, one of our ancestors' favorite superfoods.

My hope is that this book will answer all your gelatin questions and help you upgrade your health another notch.

As always, if you have additional questions, please hop over to the Facebook page and let's chat!

The Gelatin Secret 15

Most of us know gelatin as the main ingredient in Jell-O. Or, if you've ever bothered to read ingredients before, then maybe you know gelatin as the ingredient in chewy candies like Skittles and marshmallows. So, it will probably come as a surprise to hear that *real* gelatin is an incredibly nutritious food with health benefits ranging from radiant skin to improved digestion.

WHAT IS GELATIN?

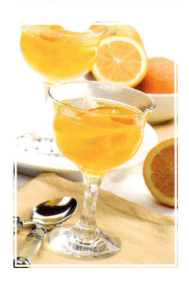

Gelatin is basically a cooked form of collagen. It is made by cooking down the bones, connective tissues, and hides of animals (which are all rich in collagen). Cooking causes the molecules of collagen to rearrange so they take on a different composition. When cool, the gelatin is firm. When warm, the gelatin melts. When mixed with water, the gelatin creates a jelly-like substance.

This leads us to the question of what is collagen. Collagen is a type of protein which is mostly found in the connective tissues of animals. It is also found in skin and is what gives our skin its elasticity, which is why collagen is touted as a natural remedy for wrinkles (You body can't absorb collagen through the skin, so forget about all of those collagen creams! You've got to eat your collagen instead. We'll get more into that later). Overall, collagen makes up about ⅓ of the protein in the human body.[1]

GLYCINE AND PROLINE: THE BASIC COMPONENTS OF COLLAGEN

The two main amino acids which make up collagen are glycine and proline and they are also found in real gelatin. Neither of these amino acids is considered "essential" because the body is capable of making them on their own. The term "non essential" is misleading though.

First off, these two amino acids *do* have essential roles in the body. It takes about 1000 amino acids to make one collagen protein in our bodies. About 33% of these amino acids are glycine, which are remarkably adept at forming tight chains. About 17% of the amino acids are proline, which twist themselves into the chains to form very tight bonds.

The unique composition and arrangement of amino acids in collagen is why collagen is so strong and dexterous.[2]

Secondly, you've got to be in good health to produce non-essential amino acids. As Vice President of the Weston A. Price Foundation Kaayla T. Daniel says of the amino acids, "Common sense suggests that the millions of Americans suffering from stiff joints, skin diseases and other collagen, connective tissue and cartilage disorders might be suffering serious shortfalls of proline, glycine and other needed nutrients."[3]

Even if you are the epitome of health and nutrition, the body still starts to produce less collagen as you get older. Without new collagen fibers being formed, the fibers in the collagen you already have become cross linked with each other, becoming rigid and stiff. This is why people typically suffer from stiff joints as they age and also why our skin loses elasticity (causing those ubiquitous wrinkles).[4]

Research shows that glycine and proline should be considered "conditionally essential" because, under most situations, the body cannot make enough of them on their own.[3] This wasn't a problem in the past when people regularly consumed broths made from the bones and connective tissues of the animals they ate. Cooking the bones helped release the collagen, which was in turn absorbed into our bodies to use for collagen production.

At least as far as collagen is concerned, we are literally what we eat.

Today, most people just consume the muscle meat of the animals they eat. While collagen makes up about 50% of the protein in animals, only about 6% of muscle tissue is collagen.[5] Muscle meat also consists of different amino acid combinations than found in collagen. As Dr. Ray Peat explains, the switch towards a muscle-meat only diet has caused a change in the amino acid profiles of our diets. We get too much of the amino acids tryptophan or cysteine (found in muscle meat), which can result in metabolic problems. By adding gelatin back into our diets, we can get back to the diet nature intended for us.[6]

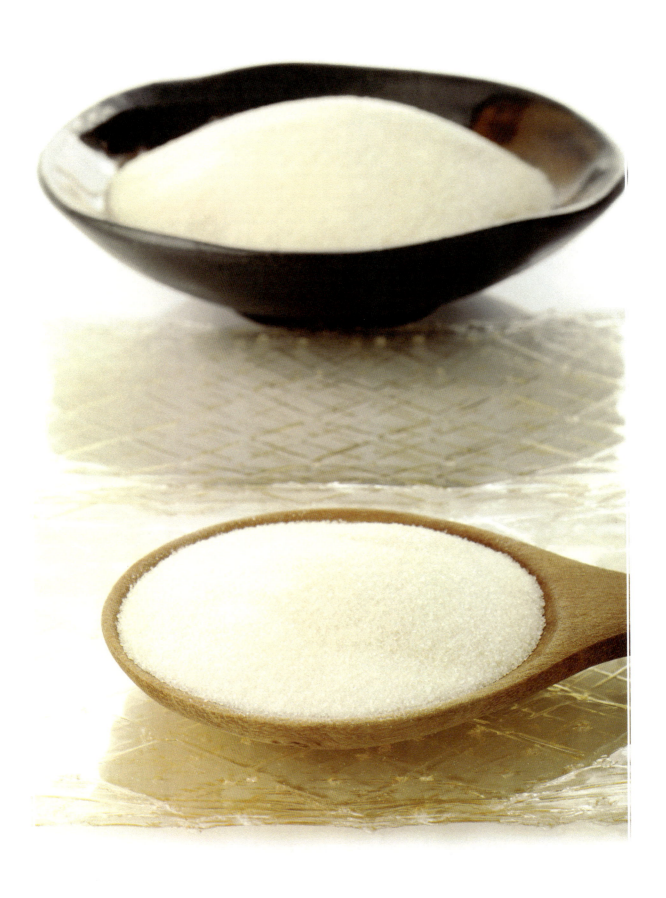

HOW IS GELATIN MADE?

> **Note:** contrary to popular belief, gelatin is NOT made from ground-up horse hooves. The hooves are very lacking in collagen.

Sorry vegetarians. This isn't for you. Gelatin is always made from animal products. Making gelatin is very simple. All you need is some animal parts which are rich in collagen. Bones are especially good, but you can also use connective tissues and skin. Gelatin can also be made from fish scales. Now, boil these parts in water for about 4+ hours.

After you are finished boiling the parts, let it cool and set for about 24 hours. The fat will drift to the top and can be skimmed off. You will be left with a gel-like substance which is the gelatin. In the 1840s, a guy named Charles Knox figured out that he could dry strips of his wife's gelatin. He then hired a team of salesmen to go door to door, showing housewives how to add water to the dried strips to get gelatin. This was the beginning of commercial gelatin. But this original commercial gelatin is a lot different than the flavorless, firm gelatin we find in today's supermarkets.

The Difference between Real Gelatin and Crap Gelatin

The gelatin that our great-great grandmothers made is a lot different than the stuff you find on supermarket shelves. I'm not even talking about all of the sugars, artificial flavorings, and other additives which go into most store-bought gelatin found in the dessert section of supermarkets. The process of how the gelatin is made completely changes its nutritional value.

Traditionally, gelatin was made from animal bones. Today, gelatin is mostly made from pig hide or, with kosher gelatin, from cow hide.[4] To help extract the collagen from the animal skin, manufacturers typically soak the hides in an acid like hydrochloric acid or calcium hydroxide. Traces of the acids remain in the gelatin and can cause health problems. In the case of the hydrochloric acid, the acid also destroys the collagen, thus destroying the nutritional benefits of the gelatin.[7]

The problem with store-bought gelatin isn't just all of the additives in it. Because it is made from one source (usually pig skin), it is lacking a full range of nutrients.

There are at least 15 different types of collagen. Different types of collagen are present in different parts of the body: the bones, skin, cartilage, ligaments, bone marrow... By consuming a gelatin made from just one part of the animal, you aren't getting the diverse types of collagen your body needs.[8]

As Dr. Kaayla Daniel from the Weston A. Price Foundation says, "As for using gelatin today for therapeutic benefits, the highest quality product would come from making gelatin at home using skins, cartilage and bones from organic chicken or meat."[3]

You will note that Dr. Daniel says the best gelatin comes from *organic* chicken or meat. This is a whole 'nother can of worms. But, in brief, I will say this: the better quality your source materials, the better quality the end product will be. Numerous studies show that animals on a natural, grass-fed diet have higher nutrient contents than factory farm animals on an unnatural grain and soy heavy diet.[9] Choosing organic, grass-fed bones for your gelatin also means that you won't have to worry about all those hormones, antibiotics and pesticides making it into your gelatin. Plus, there is also the whole ethical aspect of supporting factory farming which is destroying the environment, harming small farmers, and animal welfare…

BONE BROTH AS A SOURCE OF GELATIN

Ever wonder why chicken soup has been the go-to recipe for illnesses for centuries, earning itself names like "Jewish penicillin"? The reason is because soup made from real bone broth (I'm not talking about the crap stuff you find in a box at the store) contains high amounts of gelatin.

Now, there are a couple brands which make real gelatin from grass-fed animals (see our resource page for our recommendations). But, even these quality gelatin products don't compare to the whole caboodle that is bone broth. You can easily make bone broth at home for ridiculously cheap. If you want to save yourself the hassle and don't mind paying a bit more, there are also a few companies that sell quality ready-made broth (again, check out our recommendation on the resource page) When you cook down bones and other animal parts containing collagen, the collagen is released as gelatin. This gelatin is very rich in proline and glycine that your body can absorb.

Bones aren't just good sources of gelatin though! Broth made from bones is also rich in nutrients like calcium, phosphorus, magnesium,

HOLLYWOOD HOMESTEAD

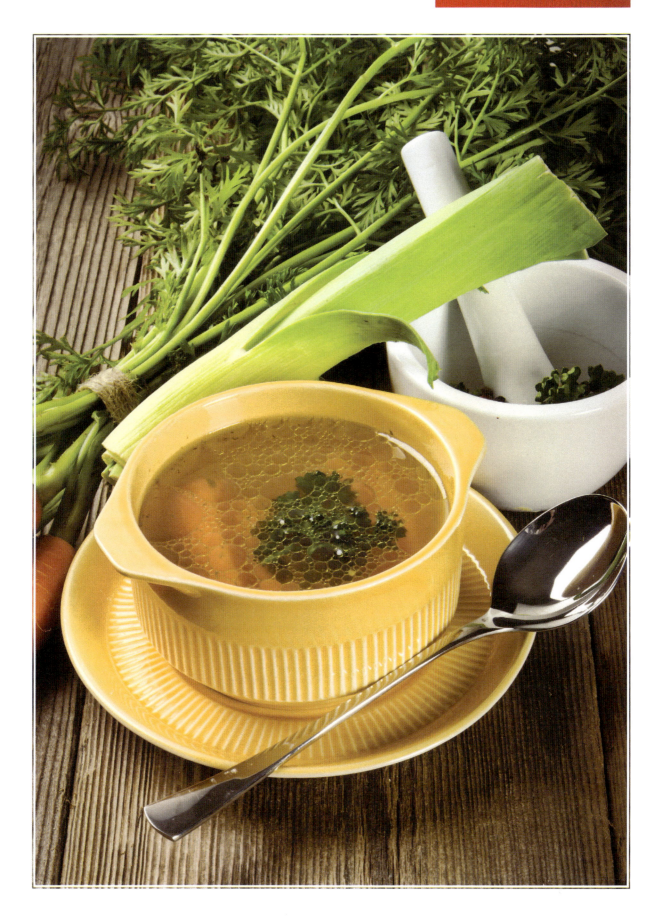

The Gelatin Secret

sulfur, and potassium. Not surprisingly, all of these are great for your bones. The bone broth itself is a liquid and rich in electrolytes, so it is also very hydrating.[10]

If you are making your bone broth from big, thick bones (as opposed to stringy chicken legs and whatnot), then your broth will also be a good source of bone marrow. Bone marrow is a superfood in its own right and books could certainly be written about all of its health benefits. It contains very high amounts of vitamins, minerals, essential fatty acids, and alkylglycerols lipids which assist in white blood cell production. It is especially good for the immune system because it transports oxygen to cells. No wonder that bone marrow is considered a delicacy in so many cultures![11, 12, 13]

Making bone broth is easy. We'll go over it in detail later in our Guide to Making Gelatin-Rich Bone Broth.

How to Get the Most from Gelatin

Ideally, we'd all consume a few cups of homemade bone broth every day. The broth would provide us with a healthy dosage of gelatin along with the many other nutrients from the bones. I've personally come to enjoy sipping on a warm cup of bone broth. If you aren't up to chugging bone broth (even a few sips would be beneficial), there are all sorts of creative ways to get it into your diet. Aside from the obvious one of making soup, you can use it to:

- steam veggies
- cook your grains in, if you eat grains
- add to sauces or just about any place you'd use water to cook with

If you can't get bone broth into your diet, then there are a couple brands which make a high-quality gelatin from pastured animals. (see our resource page). Check out the recipes section of this book to get all sorts of great ideas on how to use gelatin (family approved!). If you absolutely don't like the idea of cooking with gelatin or don't have time, there are some beef gelatin pills you can take as a supplement, like the ones on the resource page.

When consuming gelatin for health benefits, there are a couple things you need to keep in mind though:

1. Try not to microwave it

Don't heat or cook your gelatin in the microwave. Microwaving causes the proline in gelatin to change into a "cis amino acid" called *d-proline*. According to information at the Weston A. Price Foundation, cis amino acids may be hazardous to the body because they cause structural and immunological changes to peptides and proteins. Further, d-proline is toxic and can damage the liver, kidneys, and nervous system![3]

2. Take on an empty stomach or with meat

Ideally, you should consume gelatin with meat. This helps balance out the amino acid profiles of the gelatin with that of the muscle meat. Alternatively, you can take gelatin on an empty stomach. This has shown to promote Human Growth Hormone production—you know, that hormone which everyone is lining up to get shots of because it makes us look younger, boosts metabolism, and helps weight loss.[14]

Okay, these are just the *ideal* ways to consume gelatin so you get the most out of it. But simply consuming gelatin is going to do you a world of good, so don't hesitate to eat a yummy gelatin gummy snack as a dessert after your dinner.

WHY EAT GELATIN?

Aside from the nutritional value of gelatin, there are many other reasons for eating gelatin or gelatin-rich bone broth.

The Ethics of Eating Nose-to-Tail

As a former lifelong vegetarian, in addition to the digestive hurdles I had to get over when I started consuming meat again, there were some ethical hurdles as well. It was hard enough for me to wrap my head around the idea of eating a burger or a steak. The idea of eating organ meats, skin, connective tissue and every last other bit of the animal is not something that made me immediately jump for joy. But, from a logical standpoint, ironically, it is almost a commitment I felt I *had* to make. In other words, it didn't feel ethically right to be a "steak only" beef eater, or a "bacon only" pork eater. What happens to the rest of the animal? I felt a sense of responsibility to consume *all of the animal* that was nourishing me and my family.

I began purchasing our meat directly from a local farmer. At first, I bought many pounds of ground beef since it was affordable and something I knew how to cook. Eventually we found ourselves purchasing a whole cow at a time, with fat and bones included of course.

Perhaps it's a remnant from growing up in a third world country (Argentina), but I absolutely hate waste. The fact that I can make broth out of parts of the animal that are too tough for us humans to otherwise eat and digest gives me great joy. Boiling those bones down to just about nothing is the least I can do to make use of every bit of food I am lucky enough to have available for my family and me.

If you're interested in exploring this idea further, the book *Beyond Bacon* by Stacy Toth and Matthew McCarry is chock full of recipes that respect the whole hog. I also love the incredibly beautiful and useful video called *The Anatomy of Thrift* by Farmstead Meatsmith found here: http://anatomyofthrift.com/

HOLLYWOOD HOMESTEAD

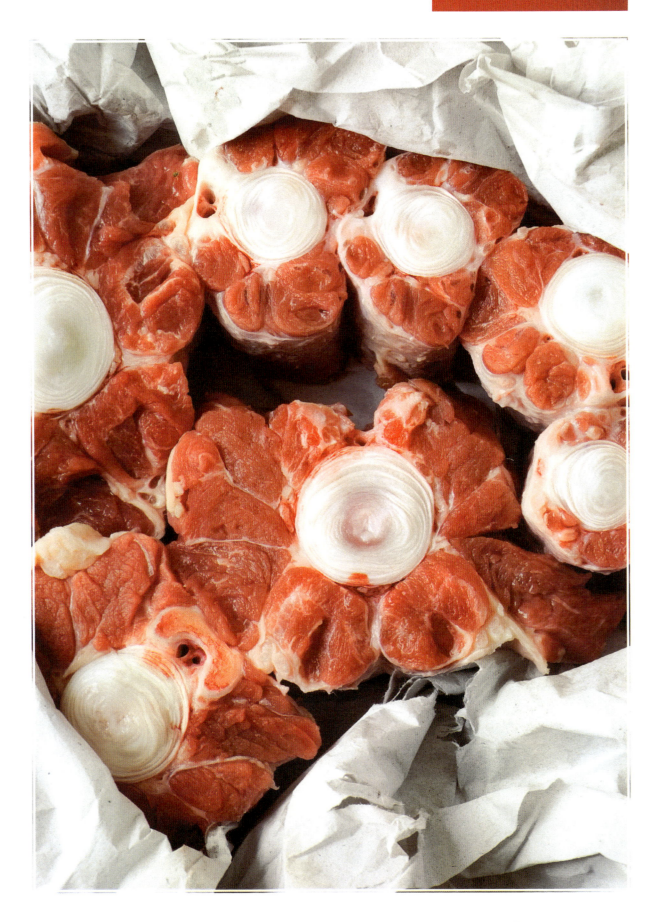

The Gelatin Secret · 25

Affordability

One of the common reasons for avoiding a healthy diet and sticking to the drive thru is that pastured meat and organic vegetables can be costly for people. I have a family of 5 and only one of us brings home a paycheck so trust me, I get it. Consuming bone broth and gelatin is one of the best things you can do to stretch your grocery budget. You'll get a lot of "bang for your buck" from a few dollars worth of healthy bones that you can cook the heck out of till they fall apart, getting several batches of broth out of one batch of bones.

Grass fed gelatin powder may seem expensive, but once you realize how little of it you need to use and how powerful its healing properties are, you'll realize you're better off cutting corners in other areas because, bite-for-bite and calorie-for-calorie, gelatin is one of the most nutrient dense and inexpensive foods you can get your hands on.

HOW TO CHOOSE GELATIN

If you are terribly industrious, you can try your hand at making gelatin powder at home. Let me warn you though: you will probably be disappointed. Homemade gelatin tastes like bones (that shouldn't come as too big of a surprise). It also won't be as firm as the gelatin you are used to because you probably lack the tools to extract all the fat and liquid from the gelatin. Don't worry though. There are a couple brands of great quality gelatin which you can buy, like the ones listed on the [resource page](). On the resource page, we've also listed one good beef gelatin supplement for those who don't have time to cook or are simply adverse to the idea of eating gelatin.

Types of Gelatin

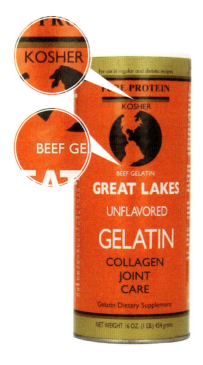
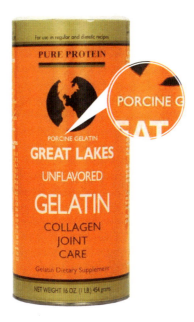
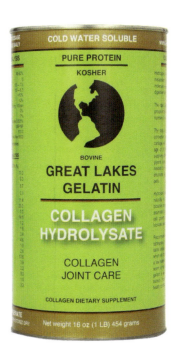

Gelatin (The red and orange canisters):

This is simply cooked collagen (the same which you would find in a homemade bone broth) which has been dried and turned into a powder. It will form a gel when mixed with water and is great for making jelly treats. **It must be mixed with warm water or else clumps will form.** Great Lakes makes two types of gelatin: Porcine (which is from pigs that may not be eating a 100% natural diet but is the cheaper option) and Kosher (which is from 100% grass-fed cows).

Collagen Hydrolysate (the green canister)

This is cooked collagen which has been heated to higher temperatures and then treated with enzymes. The process breaks the bonds between the amino acids (though keeps the amino acids themselves intact). The collagen is then turned into a dry powder. **It will NOT gel and can dissolve into both cool and warm liquids.** So, you can mix it into anything from your morning tea or coffee to mashed yams. Because the amino acid bonds are broken down, it is easier to digest, is absorbed by the body faster, and is good for people with digestion problems.

Bottom line:

For jello, gummy bears and anywhere you want it to gel, use the red one. For anything you'd like to simply sneak it into without it gelling (like smoothies or in your tea or coffee) use the green one.

HOW GELATIN NOURISHES EACH PART OF YOUR BODY

Before getting into all the specific ways gelatin can benefit your body, I want to preface it with an important note. When I refer to gelatin as a superfood I do so cautiously, because I don't want to give the impression that you can carry on eating a diet devoid of nutrients, cutting corners on sleep and carrying on through life as a ball of stress and expect gelatin to save you from the daily assault on your body. Gelatin is an amazing complement to your healthy diet and lifestyle and, while you will see some benefit from incorporating it into your diet regardless of what the rest of your plate looks like, I highly recommend you consider adopting a diet based on real foods in order to supercharge your health.

What are real foods?

Real food is food that is grown in the ground or roams the earth, that is minimally processed and not packaged in a box or bag with a shelf life of practically forever. Real food is *nutrient dense* food; food our ancestors would have recognized. By eating real foods, you are also crowding out poor-nutrient, pro-inflammatory foods like processed flours and sugars. Real food is anti-inflammatory, hence the incredible results with a paleo diet (especially a paleo autoimmune protocol) in people with autoimmune and other diseases.

My family and I follow a Paleo diet 90% of the time, although we include white rice and other gluten-free grains on occasion.

HOLLYWOOD HOMESTEAD

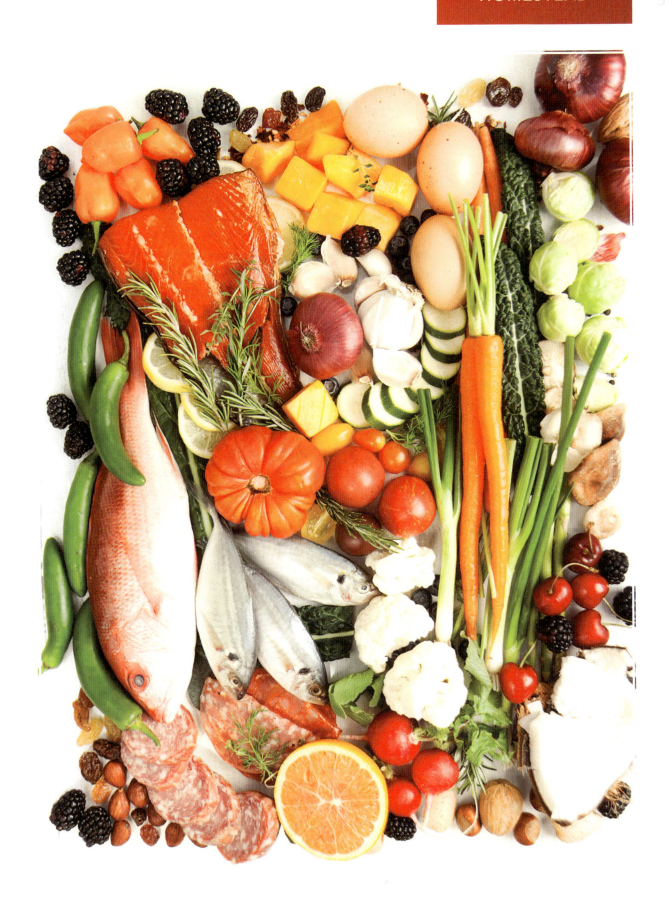

The Gelatin Secret   29

What do you eat on a Paleo diet?

Eat:

- Meat of all kinds (preferably pastured)
- Fish (preferably wild caught)
- Eggs (preferably pastured)
- Vegetables (preferably local, seasonal and organic)
- Fat, yes even saturated fat (from pastured animals, avocados, coconut, etc.)
- Fermented foods and beverages
- Fruit (preferably local, seasonal and organic)
- Nuts and seeds (if you tolerate them well)

Don't eat:

- Grains (especially gluten containing grains like wheat, rye and barley)
- Legumes (including peanuts)
- Processed foods
- Refined sugar
- Alcohol

Other real food approaches to diet which are similar to Paleo are Primal (which includes raw grass-fed dairy), and the Weston A. Price Diet (which includes raw grass-fed dairy and soaked and fermented grains). All of these approaches would fall under the category of "ancestral" or "traditional".

Eating real food might seem daunting at first, but it doesn't have to be incredibly expensive or time consuming. Just doing the best you can within your available time and budget is a great start. For more tips on how to get started with a real food approach, visit my blog at www.hollywoodhomestead.com or check out my first eBook *Paleo Made Easy* at www.thepaleosurvivalguide.com.

As important as diet is, sorry to break it to you but, even a real foods diet isn't going to be a cure-all. I can't emphasize enough the importance of stress management, getting enough sleep, and exercise. All of these go hand in hand and affect each other. Your body uses exercise to counter the effects of stress hormones. Without enough exercise, you will feel stressed and probably have a hard time sleeping. Stress, lack of exercise and poor nutrition negatively affect sleep. When you get insufficient sleep, your ability to handle everyday stressors and resist sugar cravings are impeded. It's a vicious cycle that ends with a negative impact to just about all of our systems.

> *If you want to be healthy, you can't just make one small change and expect everything to be fine. You've got to look at the bigger picture.*

SECTION 03

Gelatin for Bone Health

Since gelatin is made from bones, it shouldn't come as a surprise that gelatin is incredibly good for your bones. We tend to think of bones as the hard, inert things made of calcium which give our bodies structure. Really, bones are living tissues with marrow at its center. They are constantly being depleted and replenished and, low and behold, they are mostly made of collagen and not calcium (remember, gelatin is just a cooked form of collagen)!

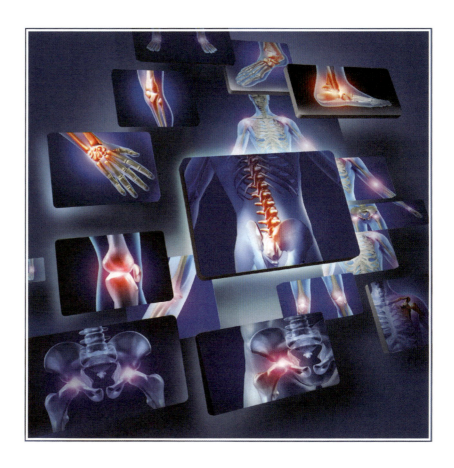

WHAT ARE BONES?

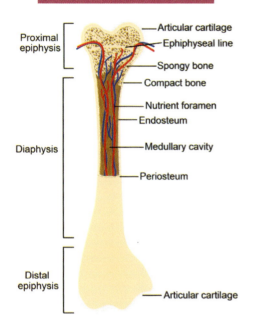

Bones are mostly made up of collagen, which is a type of protein. About 90 to 95% of bone is made of collagen.[15] So, why is it that we associate bones with calcium? Because calcium is what combines with the collagen to make bones strong. The calcium also makes the bones hard, but the collagen still makes bones a bit flexible so they can withstand stress. Over 99% of the calcium in the body is stored in bones and teeth.[16] You can think of bones as a sponge made of protein cells into which minerals are embedded and stored.

The bones we are born with are not the same bones we have throughout our lives. Rather, bone tissue renews itself in what is known as "remodeling". The first part of remodeling involves *resorption* — the process of bone tissue breaking down and being removed. The second part of remodeling involves the formation of new bone tissue. Cells called osteoclasts are in charge of resorption. Cells called osteoblasts are in charge of making new bone tissue and then they become bone cells, which can then be broken down by the osteoclasts. This process is constantly occurring, which is what allows bones to heal themselves after a fracture.[17]

When we are young, bone formation usually occurs faster than bone resorption. Obviously, adequate supplies of calcium and protein are crucial for developing healthy bones, but other nutrients are also important. Vitamin D is imperative for calcium absorption. In fact, if your calcium levels and vitamin D levels are both low, often simply taking a vitamin D supplement will take care of regulating your calcium levels as well. Vitamin K2 (which is abundant in Natto, egg yolk, full fat grass fed dairy products, pastured chicken liver, chicken breast and grass fed ground beef) helps take calcium to where it needs to go.[18] There are also many hormones which play an important role in bone formation and breakdown.

As we age, bone formation occurs more slowly. Around the age of 30, most people reach the peak of their bone formation. At this point, they start losing bone tissue faster than they form it. For women, the risk of losing too much bone tissue is especially high during menopause. This is because estrogen plays a role in bone formation and the sudden drop in estrogen levels can lead to severe bone loss, which is why osteoporosis is such a big concern for older women.[19]

WHY SUPPLEMENTS AREN'T THE BEST SOLUTION

Unfortunately, these vital bone nutrients are often lacking in the Standard American Diet (SAD). So what? People can just take supplements, right? In fact, calcium supplements were recommended for women to prevent bone loss during menopause and, based on this recommendation, surveys found that *60% of women over 60 were taking a calcium supplement.* So it must have come as a shock when the report came out showing that *calcium supplements increase the risk of heart attack by 30%!* Calcium supplements also increased risk of other cardiovascular problems and problems like kidney stones.[20,21]

Calcium supplements aren't the best solution because *it isn't always about quantity.* It is all about *getting the right balance.* Your body also needs "tools" like vitamins and minerals to use calcium properly. In the case with calcium supplements and heart disease, the calcium was getting into the blood but, without enough vitamin K2 to transport the calcium where it needed to go, it was just hardening in the arteries instead of making it to bone. Along with nutrition, other cofactors for bone health include balanced blood sugar levels and exercise.[22]

When you eat a real foods diet (which includes eating an animal nose-to-tail), you are going to get a balance of all the nutrients you need for bone health.

A perfect example of this are the fat soluble vitamins A, D, E and K2 which, when consumed in food like grass-fed beef liver, are found in perfectly-balanced proportions to one another.

COMMON BONE PROBLEMS AND DISEASES

Osteoporosis is the most well-known and talked-about condition affecting the bones, but there are numerous bone disorders affecting Americans. According to one study, 1.5 million people in the US suffer a fracture due to bone disease annually. In fact, by the time they are 50, 39.7% of women and 13.1% of men will have had a fracture.[23] The scary thing is that the number of fractures is expected to rise. From 1990 to 2050, the rate of *hip fracture* (not including other types of fractures!) is expected to go up 240% for women and 310% for men.[24]

There are all sorts of reasons why bone disease occur—such as genetics, viruses, and aging. However, with all of the major bone diseases afflicting Americans, nutrition is a key component. Considering how big of a problem bone disease is in the western world, you'd think health experts would put more emphasis on nutrition aside from their basic recommendations of taking a supplement.

Let's take a look at the main bone diseases afflicting Americans and what causes them.

Osteoporosis and Osteopenia:

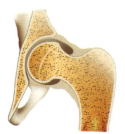

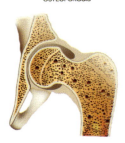

Osteoporosis is a condition which occurs when bone loss outpaces bone growth, resulting in a loss of bone density. In fact, osteoporosis literally means "porous bones". People with osteoporosis are at risk of fractures. And because their bone loss is outpacing their bone growth, it is difficult for them to recover from these fractures. Osteopenia is also a loss of bone density, but not to the degree of osteoporosis.[25]

Yes, it is "normal" for bone growth to slow down as you age, but it should never be considered normal for bone loss to outpace growth. Nutrition is the most important factor for preventing bone loss (exercise is also important). So long as your body has the nutrients it needs, then your bones will have the building blocks they need for bone growth. Gelatin helps because it provides the body with collagen it can use for building bone. Gelatin also helps improve gut health so your body is better able to absorb the other nutrients needed for bone growth, like calcium and vitamins D and K2.

Scoliosis:

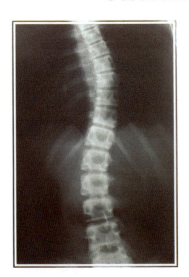

Scoliosis is a condition in which the spine curves. 85% of cases, including that of my oldest daughter, are considered "idiopathic", meaning that the cause is unknown. Scoliosis definitely has a genetic component, but there are environmental triggers as well.

Numerous studies have found that scoliosis can be induced in animals by creating deficiencies of nutrients like copper, vitamin B, and manganese. Other studies have also found that pesticides found in food can cause scoliosis in animals.[26, 27]

Even though these scientific studies don't positively link scoliosis to nutrition and nutritional deficiencies in humans, I find it interesting that my daughter who had severe scoliosis was also deficient in the fat soluble vitamins which contribute to proper bone formation: vitamins A, D and K2. Even when supplementing her with these vitamins, we realized she had a difficult time absorbing them, requiring a focus on restoring gut health.

Scoliosis is also linked to weak or loose ligaments which are unable to hold the spine in place. As we will talk about in the Gelatin for Joint Health section, getting adequate amounts of collagen is crucial for keeping your ligaments strong and healthy.[28]

Scoliosis is a problem which we mostly associate with children. However, adults can also get scoliosis. Late-onset scoliosis is linked to osteoporosis. Considering how big of a problem osteoporosis is, adults should also be worried about scoliosis as well.[29]

Rickets (Osteomalacia):

Rickets, a condition in which children's bones become weak, sounds like one of those diseases of the past which we've overcome. But it turns out that rickets is actually on the rise again. Rickets is a condition in which the bones have enough collagen but not enough minerals, so they become soft. Some of the symptoms of rickets are bowed legs, dental problems, and tender bones.

Most cases of rickets are caused by vitamin D deficiency. Without enough vitamin D, the body is unable to absorb calcium.[30] Experts theorize that rickets is on the rise again because youth today spend so much time indoors (probably playing games on the internet) instead of getting vitamin D outdoors from sunlight. Also, there are probably few youngsters who are eating natural food sources of vitamin D, like salmon and tuna.[31] Okay, gelatin isn't going to help you with your vitamin D — but it is important for overall bone health and, since it is a gut healer, it also helps you absorb the vitamins and minerals you consume better.

THE IMPORTANCE OF COLLAGEN FOR BONE HEALTH

We are usually advised to get enough calcium if we want to keep our bones healthy and strong. Ironically, no one seems to mention the importance of collagen for bone health, despite the fact that bones are mostly made up of collagen. More specifically, the type of bone cells responsible for bone formation (osteoids) are about 94% collagen.[32]

Gelatin is one of the best ways to get bioavailable forms of collagen your body needs. Studies have found that our bodies readily absorb the collagen from gelatin[33,34]. Since the amino acids in gelatin are already broken down, gelatin is a better source of collagen than foods which contain collagen.[35]

Unfortunately, there haven't been too many studies on gelatin and bone mass. However, the studies which have been done are positive (which isn't too surprising considering our bones are mostly made of collagen). One study found that hydrolyzed collagen (which is gelatin that has been heated to a higher temperature and treated with enzymes so it doesn't congeal[36]) increased bone mass in exercising rats.[37] In a study performed on humans, it was found that hydrolyzed collagen increased bone mass density when given to patients.[38] An older study found that hydrolyzed collagen triggers the formation of new collagen by attracting fibroblasts.[35]

Bone broth is even better for maintaining your bone health. This is because it also contains many of the minerals you need for healthy bones, like calcium and magnesium. It also contains high amounts of other amino acids which are important for bone health. For example, bone broth contains the amino acid lysine which helps calcium absorb into bones and aids in tissue regeneration.[39]

GELATIN FOR HEALING BONES

It is really sad that when we are healing from bone problems like fractures or breaks, all we are told to do is "take it easy". While I wouldn't advise running a marathon during this time, there are certainly a lot of proactive things we can do to speed the healing of our bones—with nutrition being the key focus.

When my daughter was recovering from major scoliosis surgery, I wasn't just about to sit back helplessly. I spent hundreds of hours researching what I could do to help her body repair itself. I credit real foods with a focus on nutrient density and supplementing with a lot of bone broth and gelatin for her recovery which was so speedy that it shocked the doctors and nurses.

While in the hospital, I offered her gelatin several times a day as well as homemade bone broth to drink in the form of soups. I also gave her avocado (rich in fat-soluble vitamins) to go along with the bland chicken breast she was being served. The doctors were impressed at how quickly she was able to lift herself out of bed. Coincidence? I think not!

Stages of Bone Healing

There are three different stages of bone healing. Gelatin can help with *all* of these stages.

- **Initial Stage:** The first stage of bone healing is inflammation. When a bone fractures, the blood vessels also break. A clot is formed at the breaking point. The purpose of the clot is to cut off blood flow to the damaged bone edges. The clot also keeps the bone pieces lined up. Without blood flowing to the fracture, the damaged bone cells quickly die off. Osteoclast cells come to carry away the dead bone tissue and recycle it into new tissue. Inflammation occurs as the cells do their work.

- **Reparative Stage:** Now, repair cells come to the fracture site. They develop into specialized cells which form new bone. Among them are chondrocytes which release collagen and proteoglycans. These cells form together to make a soft callus around the fracture site. The soft callus is still fragile, which is why you are supposed to "take it easy" during this stage. The body then releases minerals like calcium into the soft callus which weave the tissue together, hardening the callus.

- **Remodeling Stage:** The hard callus now begins the process of remodeling. This can take months or years as the callus is broken down by osteoclast cells and new bone is formed by osteoblast cells. The bone eventually regains its original shape.[39,40,41]

During the initial stage, gelatin can help by soothing inflammation. Now, keep in mind that inflammation is important to the healing process, but it is also very painful. Medications like NSAIDs (Non steroidal anti-inflammatory drugs) are often used to control the pain, but they actually block the acute inflammation process (which is necessary and normal when recovering from injury or surgery!), which means that healing takes longer. By nourishing your body with foods that naturally reduce inflammation (including gelatin as well as nutrients like vitamin C, bioflavonoids, and Omega 3 fatty acids), you relieve painful inflammation while speeding healing.[39]

As a source of protein, gelatin can also be incredibly important for speeding up the reparative stage. Protein boosts insulin-like growth factor-1 (IGF-1) which helps the process of renewing bone, boosting immune response, and skeletal rigidity. Without enough protein during the bone repairing stage, a rubbery callus will form instead of a strong, rigid one. Since collagen is one of the main components of the callus, supplementing with gelatin is a good way to help with callus formation.[39]

As we talked about earlier, the osteoblast cells which are responsible for remodeling bones are primarily made up of collagen. So, it isn't too surprising that multiple studies show that supplementing with collagen helps the bone remodeling process by stimulating osteoblast cells.[42]

Considering all of this, it makes sense that gelatin is one of the standard foods you will find in a hospital. Too bad they use the crap brands of gelatin and not the grass-fed varieties which are sourced from bones and not just hide! (Read about The Difference between Real Gelatin and Crap Gelatin) The quality of gelatin is imperative to the success of your recovery. Smuggle it into the hospital from home and toss the hospital gelatin in the trash where it belongs!

Gelatin for Joint Health

Many people assume that joint pain is a normal part of the aging process. Yes, joint pain may be common — but that does not mean it should be considered normal! Joint pain is a sign that your body is suffering and unable to heal itself.

According to one survey, 19% of Americans have chronic joint pain and 84% of them were taking over-the-counter drugs for the pain.[43] Another survey found that about ⅓ of US adults had suffered from some joint pain in the past month.[44] Obviously, we've got an epidemic joint problem on our hands which "aging" alone doesn't explain.

WHAT ARE OUR JOINTS MADE OF?

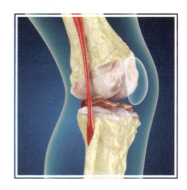

A joint is all of the parts around where two or more bones meet so those bones can move. There are four main tissues which make up joints.

- **Cartilage**: covers the ends of bones to cushion them; is slippery to reduce friction during movement

- **Capsule**: surrounds the bones to prevent them from moving too much

- **Ligament**: holds the joint together

- **Muscle**: muscles are attached to the joint by tendons and move the bones

The connective tissues in our joints are primarily made up of collagen. Now, this is a pretty vague statement since there are so many types of collagen. Dr. Kaayla Daniel explains it very well in her famous article "Why Broth is Beautiful"[3]. She researched why glycine and proline (the main components of the collagen in our body as well as gelatin) are so important for joint health.

According to her research, cartilage in the human body gets its strength from a network of criss-crossing collagen fibers. The network is very dense yet is ultimately a gel, which is why cartilage is so flexible.

Glycine is the main amino acid in the network. It is very small and can form into very dense chains. Proline and hydroxyproline (another major amino acid in gelatin) twist themselves into helixes around the glycine to make tight, rod-like molecules. The result is a highly structured complex chain of proteins which is very strong and flexible.

Special cells called chondrocytes live in cartilage tissue. Their job is to make *proteoglycan* molecules. These molecules are "very thirsty" and absorb lots of water, thus keeping the cartilage lubricated. The chondrocyte cells also regulate cartilage metabolism and are responsible for building new cartilage when needed. And what do they use to build new cartilage? The very same amino acids that make up collagen and cartilage: proline and glycine.

Without enough proline and glycine, our bodies won't be able to produce new cartilage. It is true that our bodies can produce proline and glycine on their own (which is why they are considered "inessential"). However, Dr. Daniel states that this is probably only true of people who are in good health. She goes on to say that, "Common sense suggests that the millions of Americans suffering from stiff joints, skin diseases and other collagen, connective tissue and cartilage disorders might be suffering serious shortfalls of proline, glycine and other needed nutrients."

THE PROOF IS IN THE (GELATIN) PUDDING

The health benefits of gelatin for joint health is one area which has been extensively studied (and not just by Nabisco in attempt to sell more of their Knox gelatin products!). Not too surprisingly, the evidence shows that consuming gelatin can increase the amount of cartilage in the joints of animals. Rebuilding cartilage is a slow process though as only some of the consumed gelatin gets added to collagen tissues. So, you can't just take a shot of gelatin and expect to heal your joints overnight. But, gelatin *can* produce relief from joint pain almost immediately.[6,45]

Now, there are a lot of different types of arthritis (over 100!). The most common one is osteoarthritis, or "wear and tear arthritis", and occurs when joint tissue gets worn down. The next big one is rheumatoid arthritis, which is an autoimmune disease in which your body attacks its own joints.[46] Now, keep in mind that arthritis is just a blanket term

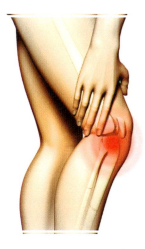

for inflammation in the joints. Regardless of the type of arthritis, gelatin can help by reducing inflammation.

Glycine has very strong immunosuppressive effects (meaning it will stop the inflammation response).[47] Reports show that it can provide the same level of relief as anti-inflammatory pills or cortisol.[45] That is sort of mind blowing isn't it?

Gelatin can also combat the inflammation of arthritis because it balances out your amino acid intake. Muscle meats contain high amounts of tryptophan, an excitatory amino acid which in excess can cause muscle pain. Glycine is an inhibitory amino acid and balances the effects of tryphtophan.[6]

Since gelatin is so nutritious and actually helps build healthy joints, which would you rather take: non steroidal anti-inflammatory drugs (NSAIDs) like ibuprofen which only temporarily provide relief of the *symptoms*, or would you rather take gelatin, the very thing that your body needs to rebuild your disintegrating joints while providing immediate relief from inflammation and long-term benefits by treating the *root of the problem*? Gelatin 1, NSAIDs 0.

If you are getting your gelatin from bone broth (which we discussed on page 20), then you are doing your joints even more good. Bone broth contains high amounts of glucosamine and chondroitin, two of the very supplements which are commonly used for relieving joint pain.[48]

GELATIN + VITAMIN C FOR HEALTHY JOINTS

So far, we've talked a lot about the amino acid glycine which is found in gelatin for joint health. But the other major amino acid in gelatin, proline, is also incredibly important for healthy joints. About 15% of collagen is comprised of proline. It is what gives collagen its stability. Further, proline is needed for collagen production.[49]

For a long time, proline didn't get a lot of attention because our bodies can make it out of the amino acid glutamic acid. Glutamic acid is readily found in many foods, including all meats, eggs, and dairy products, so proline deficiency was presumably rare. However, sometimes the problem isn't the absence of proline but rather not having enough vitamin C.

The Gelatin Secret

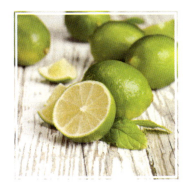

Vitamin C is needed to turn proline into a different form called *hydroxyproline*. This is the active form of the proline which our bodies use to make collagen. So, it isn't enough just to get proline in your diet. You also need to make sure your body has enough vitamin C in order to turn proline into hydroxyproline.

Hydroxyproline is also found in elastin. Elastin is like collagen in that it is a protein found in connective tissues and your skin. However, it has a different composition of amino acids and has protein sequences that process hormonal activity. As the name implies, it is very elastic and is what makes your skin bounce back into place after you pull it.[50]

Have you heard of the disease scurvy which occurs because of vitamin C deficiency? One of the symptoms of scurvy is gum disease and loosened teeth. This is because the vitamin C deficiency was preventing collagen synthesis and collagen is crucial for gum and dental health (more on that later in the Gelatin for Dental Health section).

To make sure that your body is utilizing the proline in gelatin, you will want to make sure you are consuming enough vitamin C along with your gelatin (like in the Lemon Gummies recipe). But there is more. Iron and biotin are also important cofactors for turning proline into hydroxyproline.[3,51]

This goes to show it isn't enough to take a supplement which contains just the one nutrient you think you need. Without the full spectrum of supporting vitamins and minerals, your body won't be able to make use of that nutrient. This is why it is best to get your nutrients from *real foods* which contain a variety of nutrients. So go ahead and cook yourself a nice pot of comforting soup using bone broth and you are on your way to a healthier life.

Gelatin for Gut Health

If you only read one section in this eBook, please, let it be this one. The truth is that healing your gut can be the answer to most of your problems.

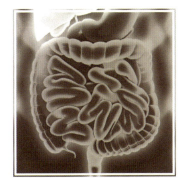

Compared to other organs like our hearts, the gut gets really little attention. This is unfortunate because digestive health is linked to everything including weight, energy, nutrition, and immunity.[52]

It isn't just what we put into our mouths which counts. The ability of our digestive system to break down and absorb these nutrients makes it or breaks it when it comes to supporting every organ and system in our body. Eating food *stuff* (highly processed junk like Twinkies) instead of real food sets our guts up for a challenge. There's not much, if any, nutrition to extract from junk food and our bodies have to constantly defend themselves from the onslaught of difficult-to-break-down, hard to recognize particles.

Our gut is like the portal to the rest of our body. It is the first line of defense where damaging particles, bad bacteria, toxins and waste can be handled and eliminated before contaminating and damaging the rest of the body. If that first line of defense is damaged and asleep at the wheel, other organs and systems will be affected and will have to step up to fight.

WHAT IS LEAKY GUT SYNDROME?

Our guts are designed to allow only *fully broken-down* proteins (that are now amino acids) to pass through the intestinal walls and into our bloodstream so they can be used by the body. The problem is that the gut can get damaged and gaps can form in the lining (aka leaky gut syndrome). When this happens, partially undigested particles of food and toxins that were supposed to be eliminated will get into the bloodstream. When the immune system gets wind of this, it attacks these foreign invaders to handle the problem. This is normally great but, in the case of leaky gut, there are a lot of foreign invaders and they are constantly coming. The immune system is chronically on hyper-alert mode and this, over time, leads to chronic inflammation.

I like how Sean Croxton of UndergroundWellness.com describes gut permeability by comparing it to a window screen. The small holes in the screen let air pass through but keep gnats and flies outside. If the window screen gets damaged though, those invaders can get inside. In this example, the screen is the lining of the gut, the gnats and flies are undigested food particles and toxins, and the air is the amino acids our bodies need.

Here is where things get worse. A lot of those undigested particles resemble parts of our own bodies. Your overworked immune system can't tell the difference between the invaders and your own tissue! This triggers an autoimmune response in which your body attacks itself.[53]

Leaky gut syndrome is one of the requirements for all autoimmune diseases to develop and many people suffering from autoimmune diseases have reversed them by focusing on repairing their leaky guts.[54] Yes, you read that correctly:

ALL AUTOIMMUNE DISEASES START WITH LEAKY GUT.

It is not surprising that some predict that leaky gut will soon become the #1 killer in America.[55] If you have an autoimmune disease, you'll likely always have some degree of leaky gut. However, focusing on repairing your gut is imperative to keep your disease under control. At the very minimum, this can keep it from progressing and may even put it into remission.

WHAT MAKES A GUT BECOME LEAKY?

So what causes a gut to become permeable anyway? Food sensitivities are the big culprit here, with a big finger pointing to gluten; you know, the protein in wheat, barley, rye and a few other grains. In a Standard American Diet (SAD), it would not be uncommon to have waffles or toast for breakfast, a sandwich for lunch and pasta for dinner. Besides not being the most nutrient dense menu, grains are also very inflammatory in high quantities over time.

In 2000, researchers discovered a protein in humans which controlled the gaps between villi in the gut (refresher: villi are the small, fingerlike projections that line our guts and allow particles to pass). They dubbed this protein *zonulin*.[56] They later found that gliadin (the main protein in wheat gluten) causes release of zonulin. In translation: gluten causes gaps to form in your gut lining!

Gluten isn't the only culprit which is making holes in your gut. Any food that our bodies are not able to completely digest will exist as large particles inside the gut. Pasteurized milk and excessive amounts of sugar, both staples in the SAD diet, are the big ones. Those large particles will irritate the villi, causing small tears in the lining of the gut. The undigested food particles can then escape through the tears and into your bloodstream where they don't belong.[53] This is what we refer to as **food sensitivities**.

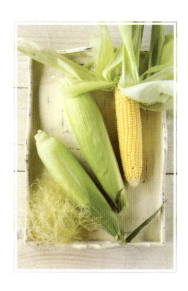

There is also ample evidence that GMOs are causing leaky gut syndrome, including studies that show toxins in GM corn can poke holes in the intestines.[57] Holes, anyone?

Antibiotics are also to blame because they kill off healthy bacteria in our guts, potentially causing harmful bacteria to flourish and inflame the gut wall. When there are more Jokers than Batmans, we end up with some serious issues! Antibiotics will also kill off the "good" bacteria in your gut which normally keep yeast in check. The yeast can then get out of control (which is why yeast infections are such a problem for people taking antibiotics). The yeast (usually candida) then grow tentacles which attach to the lining of the intestines and make holes in the lining. A diet high in sugar can also make yeast grow out of control.[58]

For all of you suffering from yeast infections, here is a cool fact: studies have found that gelatin blocks candida from adhering to certain cells types in the body![59] It still isn't clear if gelatin can fight yeast infections, but the initial studies certainly look promising.

Ironically, common over-the-counter anti-inflammatory drugs like NSAIDs (Ibuprofen for example) can also harm the gut wall because they affect gastrointestinal mucus production, making it easier for acids and enzymes to tear holes in the gut wall.[60] Anything else that causes chronic inflammation to the gut could also be to blame, like stress or excessive alcohol consumption.[61]

WHY YOU SHOULD BE WORRIED ABOUT LEAKY GUT

Let me repeat: leaky gut is the precursor to autoimmune disease! Even if you for some reason aren't worried about developing autoimmune disorders like Type I diabetes, lupus, or Multiple Sclerosis, the immediate effects of a leaky gut aren't to be taken lightly—and they are just likely to get worse.

When your gut isn't functioning properly, it can't absorb nutrients properly. So, you become tired all of the time and end up with an array of nutrient deficiencies, which can cause their own wide range of symptoms.

It's not just what you eat, it's what you absorb!

Food particles aren't the only thing that can escape through a leaky gut. Bacteria and yeast can also escape, which puts you at risk of infection. Isn't it fun to be sick all of the time?!

Remember how I said that gut health is linked to all parts of your body? Well, leaky gut syndrome sometimes doesn't show with the obvious problems like bloating and other digestive problems. It is linked to mood problems (including depression), skin problems, obesity, allergies, diabetes, and the list goes on—and this is all before you've developed a full-blown autoimmune disorder.[62,63]

CHRONIC INFLAMMATION = WORSENING PROBLEM

When your gut starts letting through one particle, it doesn't stop there. To fight the foreign particles in the bloodstream, the immune system triggers inflammation. The inflammation of the gut just means that the gut becomes *more leaky*. Now you've got more particles and bigger particles slipping through your gut. You develop new food sensitivities. More parts of your body become targets of your confused immune system and antigen antibody complexes get stored throughout your body. This means you get more symptoms. Suddenly, you've got asthma, lupus, or arthritis![64]

SIGNS YOU HAVE A LEAKY GUT

One common telltale sign you have leaky gut is when you are seemingly allergic to *everything*. Chances are, you are actually not. At least, you probably are not doomed to be allergic to this long list for the rest of your life because the problem is really leaky gut. Having multiple food sensitivities (which can produce allergy-like symptoms) is one of the biggest warnings signs that you've got leaky gut.[64] The good news is that, unlike allergies, those sensitivities may be reversible.

What's the Difference between a Food Allergy and Food Sensitivity?

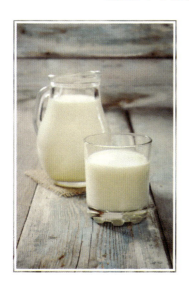

A food allergy is an allergic reaction in which your body thinks a substance which is normally harmless is something harmful. The immune system releases its soldiers (in this case, histamines) to fight off the substance. The result is a lot of inflammation and some nasty symptoms like diarrhea, rashes, and stomach ache.

Allergies are immune reactions but they are not *autoimmune* because your body is attacking the allergen and not itself.

A food sensitivity is any food which irritates the digestive tract. Milk is probably the most well-known food sensitivity but people are finally figuring out that wheat is a major irritant too. Like with a food allergy, the irritation caused by food sensitivities leads to inflammation in the digestive tract. So, a lot of the symptoms of food sensitivity are the same as allergies. It is easy to understand why we get the two confused. One of the major differences between a food allergy and sensitivity though is that the symptoms of a food allergy occur immediately (hives for example). With food sensitivity, symptoms *might* not show for a few hours or even a day (diarrhea, brain fog..). This can make it hard to pinpoint which food is causing the reaction.[65]

Note: *The terms "food sensitivity" and "food intolerance" are often used interchangeably. However, they are different in that food intolerance occurs when the body lacks an enzyme to digest a substance (such as the lactose enzyme in lactose-intolerant people). Food sensitivities can occur even when the person has enzymes which could digest the food but may be unable to do so because of other problems, such as excess consumption or a damaged gut. Both conditions have similar symptoms and can lead to gut inflammation and leaky gut.*

If you only occasionally consumed a food which irritates the digestive tract, it wouldn't be such a terrible thing because the body would have time to heal itself. I'm not saying you *should* eat foods that cause irritation, but it won't be the end of the world if you have some goat cheese as a treat every once in a while. But so many of us on today's SAD diet eat pretty much nothing but digestive irritants. Just consider all the people who eat a bagel for breakfast, a sandwich for lunch, crackers for a snack, and then top it off with a baguette with dinner. That's wheat at every meal! Now add all the other digestive irritants which are found in processed foods to the mix, such as the red dye number 40 in that cupcake you ate at a school function and you end up with a gut that is constantly inflamed.

As we talked about before, constant inflammation of the gut is going to affect the villi lining your gut. This sets off the chain reaction we talked about earlier which results in leaky gut syndrome.

HOW TO DIAGNOSE FOOD SENSITIVITIES AND LEAKY GUT SYNDROME

There are all sorts of tests to diagnose food *allergies*, like the skin prick test in which they basically rub common allergens into small wounds on your body to see if you have a reaction. With food *sensitivities* though, diagnosis methods have a long way to go.

When you have a food sensitivity, your body will produce antibodies. One option for diagnosing food sensitivity is to take a blood test which looks for antibodies associated with common food sensitivities. Cyrex Laboratories offers these tests. The tests currently cost upwards of $500 each and are usually not covered by insurance. Unfortunately, even these tests aren't always a reliable way to tell if you have a food sensitivity. They only screen for the components of foods which people usually react to and you still have to have the antibodies from that food in your body. If, for example, you've been gluten free for a few months, taking a gluten sensitivity panel might prove pointless since your test result will likely be a false negative.[66]

If you think that your food sensitivity has already developed into full-blown leaky gut syndrome, there are some diagnostic tests available. One option is a Lactulose/Mannitol test (also called Polyethelyne

Glycol test). Basically, you are given a solution made up of two different sugars. One sugar has small cells (which should be easily absorbed) and the other has large cells (which shouldn't readily pass through the gut). A urine sample is then analyzed to see the levels of these sugars. If you have high levels of both sugars in your urine, then it is a sign your gut is leaky.

Another option is a Comprehensive Stool and Digestive Analysis Test (CSDA). A stool sample is taken to look for parasites, bacteria, and yeast levels as these are indicative of gut problems. Your levels of an antibody called IgA can also be analyzed, which helps determine the condition of your gut mucosal lining. Stool tests also can look for antibodies to gliadin, the protein in gluten.[65]

Making Sense of Diagnostic Tests

There are a lot of different tests available for diagnosing specific food allergies, sensitivities, or intolerances. However, these are the most common ones you will find.

IgE Antibody Test (food allergy test)

- IgE antibodies bind themselves to the allergic food *and* a special "mast" cell. The mast cell contains histamine. When body is exposed to the allergic food again, the antibody will *instantly* create symptoms.

- IgE antibodies are primarily located in the lungs, skin, and mucus membranes and produce symptoms like hives, swelling, wheezing, rashes, diarrhea, and trouble breathing.

- Only IgE reactions are considered true allergies.

IgG Antibody Test (food sensitivity test)

- IgG antibodies bind themselves directly to the food as it enters the body and then circulate in the bloodstream. They do not bind to mast cells like IgE antibodies.

- IgG antibodies are found in *all* body fluids and can cause symptoms like migraines, irritable bowel syndrome, bloating, indigestion, and eczema.

- Symptoms can take hours or days to appear

- This is the most commonly used test for food sensitivities because the IgG antibodies are present in the body for long periods of time.

IgA Antibody Test (food sensitivity test)

- IgA antibodies are abundant in the mucus membranes of the gut and respiratory passages.

- IgA antibodies may form if the lining of the gut becomes damaged or inflamed.

- They are the only antibody that gets secreted into the digestive fluids and are thus specific to digestive problems.

- Many people (about 1 in 500) have a *deficiency* in IgA. This is considered an immune disorder and its cause is unknown, though evidence shows there is a genetic component and that stress could cause IgA deficiency. People with IgA deficiency can experience allergy-like symptoms. Low IgA is also linked to celiac disease.

- It is possible for IgG tests to be negative and IgA tests to be positive, or vica versa. The IgA test is recommended for people with suspected leaky gut syndrome

Food Intolerance Tests

- A food intolerance is when your body lacks a specific enzyme required for digesting a food, such as the lactose enzyme in lactose intolerant people. A food sensitivity is when the body negatively reacts to a food.

- Depending on the suspected intolerance, different tests may be used including hydrogen breath tests, glucose-level blood tests, and stool tests.[68, 69, 70, 71, 72]

Elimination Diet is Still the Easiest Diagnosis Method

Want a cheaper and easier way to diagnose whether you've got food sensitivities and leaky gut syndrome? An elimination diet is still the best method. This basically means you avoid certain foods for a specific period of time (usually 30 days) and see whether your symptoms improve. Then you gradually reintroduce one item at a time. If symptoms return, then that food is a culprit. Keep in mind that there can be multiple culprits, so you've got to wait until symptoms go away again before you try reintroducing another food. Granted, this won't tell whether the problem is an allergy, a food sensitivity, or leaky gut syndrome but, considering how unreliable the current diagnostic methods are, it is the best option for people who aren't in a hurry.

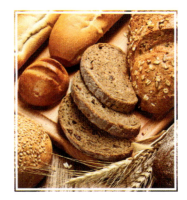

The most common culprits that you may want to consider eliminating are gluten, grains, legumes, eggs, nuts, alcohol, caffeine, nightshades, processed sugars, and processed foods. And, to be honest, the only ones worth reintroducing from a nutritional standpoint are eggs, especially the yolks since they're packed full of nutrients (and I promise they won't give you a heart attack, just stick to the pastured ones and we won't tell the doc). Nightshades and nuts you may want to try reintroducing as well simply because knowing whether or not you need to avoid them long term will give you a lot more flexibility when you're out and about eating at restaurants and traveling.

How long should the elimination diet last? It depends on how bad your symptoms are and how long it takes for you to feel benefits (assuming that your symptoms are alleviated at all). For gluten, Chris Kresser recommends avoiding it for at least 30 days before you try reintroducing it.[66] Do note that you've got to be *really* strict about sticking to the elimination diet if you want to accurately gauge your results! And with something like gluten which is a sneaky ingredient found in just about everything, a lot of label reading will be required.

HOW TO REPAIR LEAKY GUT

If you haven't already done so, the first order of business would be to eliminate the foods (or worse, food*stuff*) that damaged your gut in the first place. Eating real foods of the highest quality you can afford is the best place to start for both prevention and treatment. By "real foods", I mean food with ingredients that you could find in nature. So, none of those processed junk foods with their scientific-sounding, unpronounceable names and mass quantities of refined sugars. These foods wreak havoc on your gut, causing inflammation and upsetting the balance of your gut flora.

You'll also need to avoid foods which cause inflammation or upset the gut in other ways. This means avoiding grains. Yes, even "healthy" whole grains and also legumes (that includes peanuts). Grains and legumes are difficult to break down. They also contain chemicals like phytates which block nutrient absorption. Further, they crowd out room on your plate for more nutrient dense foods such like as pasture-raised meat and vegetables.

Ideally I would also avoid consuming large quantities of nuts as you are trying to heal your gut since they are also difficult to break down, and the goal is to make it as easy on our guts as possible, especially during this repair phase. Nuts that are soaked and dehydrated are a bit easier to digest but I would suggest avoiding them altogether or at least keeping them to a minimum until you get some repair underway.

Instead, focus on all kinds of meat (preferably pastured or wild caught) and plenty of vegetables and some fruit (preferably organic). You'll also want to make sure you are consuming probiotics to provide your body with healthy gut bacteria. Kombucha is by far my favorite probiotic (check out my recipe for Kombucha Jello!), but you can also look for (or make your own) lacto-fermented pickles, sauerkraut, beets, carrots or many other vegetables. Lacto-fermentation is the *real* way to make pickles, not like those ones you usually find in stores which are just soaked in vinegar. Real pickles will always be in the refrigerated section. In the United States, Bubbies is a good brand for fermented pickles and sauerkraut and you should be able to find them at your local grocery store. There are also other great brands popping up every day. Just check to make sure the ingredients say only *vegetable + salt*. That's it. No funny business.

If you already eat a paleo or real food diet, try taking it up a notch and focus on more nutrient dense foods such as organ meat, bone broth as often as possible, more quantity and variety of vegetables, and keeping paleo treats to a minimum. If you are coming from a SAD diet and need help getting started with a real food approach check out my website for tips and recipes www.hollywoodhomestead.com or my eBook, *Paleo Made Easy: Getting your Family Started with the Optimal Healthy Lifestyle* at www.thepaleosurvivalguide.com.

SO, WHAT DOES GELATIN HAVE TO DO WITH REPAIRING LEAKY GUT?

It turns out gelatin is one of the best foods you can eat for your gut. It basically acts like spackle and fills in holes in the gut lining. No wonder bone broth, with its high amounts of gelatin, is considered the go-to remedy for any digestive problem![55]

Aside from calming and repairing the digestive tract, gelatin can also help gut health by increasing the amount of gastric acids which are secreted. Wait, more acid? You suffer from reflux? Well, it might blow your mind to know that acid reflux is actually *caused* by not having enough acid as opposed to having too much (oh, and those antacids are not doing you any favors). Our guts need gastric acid in order to adequately break down proteins. When proteins are properly digested, they won't irritate the gut lining nor will we need to worry about big, undigested particles getting through the gut into our bloodstream.[73]

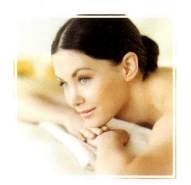

Lifestyle is also key for preventing and repairing damage to your body. Acute (once in a while and short-lived) stress is unavoidable, but the chronic (constant) stress we endure these days is very damaging to our body and hinders our efforts to repair it. Incorporating stress management techniques, sleeping at least 8 hours in a dark room and going to bed on time, meditating and taking steps to reduce stress in our day to day life is incredibly important. If your life is a ball of stress, don't panic, just take 1 step at a time to create a life that is conducive to improving and maintaining your health. Oh, and gelatin can even help you with your stress as we talk about in the Gelatin for the Brain section.

Be patient. Healing takes time and rarely happens overnight. It took years to damage your gut so it would be unreasonable to think that it could repair in a couple of months. Keeping a journal might be helpful as a way of tracking your symptoms and progress. Sometimes it's hard to notice the improvements since they are so gradual but, even if you jot down once a week, you'll have something to look back on and it can be pretty enlightening and encouraging when you look back at several weeks earlier and notice how far you've come since then.

If you want to find out more about how important your gut is for health, I strongly recommend checking out the book *Gut and Psychology Syndrome (GAPS)*. You can find it on our resource page

Gelatin for Weight Loss

No, of course I am not talking about eating sugar-free Jell-O as a way of losing weight. As a matter of fact, I'm begging you to avoid sugar-free junky Jell-O. The artificial sweeteners and flavors in those snacks are not going to do your body any good! But, by incorporating real *gelatin into your diet, you can experience some great health benefits which make weight loss easier. Here is how gelatin can help you lose weight.*

GELATIN REGULATES BLOOD SUGAR LEVELS

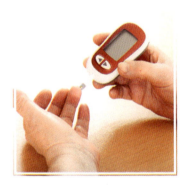

If you are trying to lose weight or just need a good reason to stay away from all that carb-laden junk food, then it is worth it to do some research into blood sugar levels and how they affect us. In a nutshell, here's the deal with blood sugar.

Your body always has some glucose (sugar) in the blood. The glucose comes from the foods you eat or from your body breaking down energy stores (like fat or muscle) to turn into glucose. The sugar provides you with energy for your brain, organs, muscles, and basic functioning. When your blood sugar levels fall below a certain level, the "hunger hormone" ghrelin is released. So, your body knows to eat some food and it turns the carbohydrates into glucose to give you more energy. Your blood sugar levels then rise and your body produces leptin, the hormone which makes you feel full.

Here is where problems start. Those of us prone to overeating or eating the super-sugary foods in the Standard American Diet (SAD) get way too much sugar at a meal. And by sugar I don't just mean that granulated white stuff. I'm also talking about things that our body sees as sugar, things that turn into sugar in our blood like bread, pasta, cereals, tons of fruit, etc. These all cause our blood sugar levels to spike. The pancreas produces insulin to deal with the sugar. It moves the excess glucose out of the blood and into storage. Now, your blood sugar levels have gone from being sky-high to crashing way down low. And what happens when you have low blood sugar levels? Your body produces the hunger hormone and you start craving sugary foods to eat.

What does all of this have to do with gelatin? It turns out that the glycine in gelatin can help regulate blood sugar levels.

Our bodies were never meant to eat a diet high in carbs. Instead, our ancestors got their energy from meat and protein. But wait, you say. Aren't carbs just sugars, and don't we need sugar for energy? Actually, our bodies can make sugar out of fat and protein using a process called *gluconeogenesis* (gluco = glucose, neo = new, genesis = making). Gluconeogenesis mainly occurs in the liver.

Today, most of us are eating way too many carbs, which means our bodies don't use fat for energy. It just sits there and eventually turns into muffin tops.

Gelatin aids in the process of gluconeogenesis. Gelatin and glycine have also been shown to facilitate the action of insulin in lowering blood sugar levels and alleviating diabetes.[74] In fact, gelatin has been used to treat diabetes for over 100 years. With the so-called "advancement" of medicine though, it seems we've largely forgotten about gelatin.[6,68]

Gelatin is by no means imperative for regulating blood sugar levels, but it can definitely help. So, if you are suffering from blood sugar problems, sugar cravings, or weight problems, it can help to include some in your diet (since gelatin is an incomplete protein, you will still need other sources of protein). You can easily add gelatin to a smoothie. There are also lots of tasty treats you can make out of gelatin, which happen to be great at quelling a sweet tooth but are low calorie so good for weight loss too. The recipe section in this eBook will get you started.

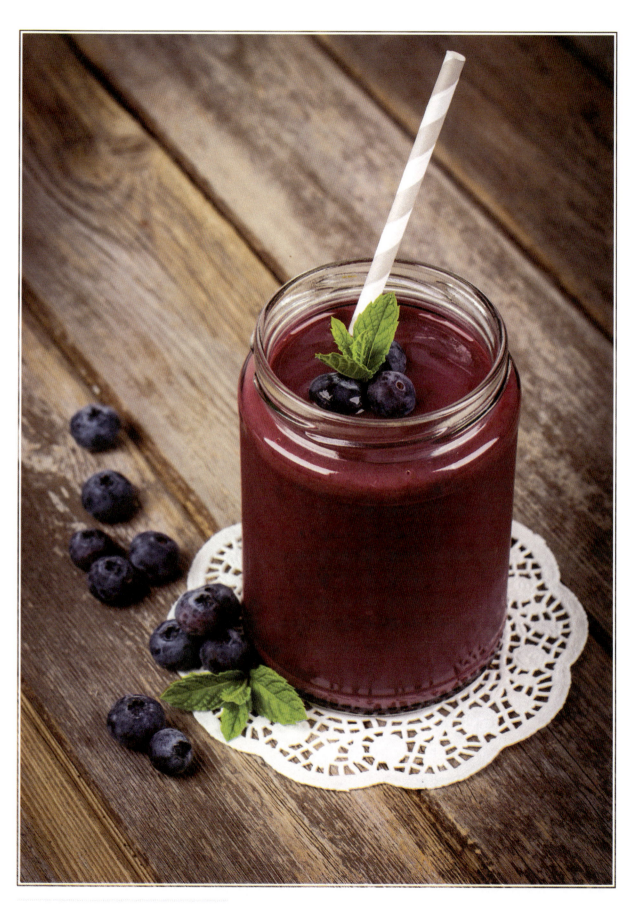

GELATIN INHIBITS SUGAR CRAVINGS

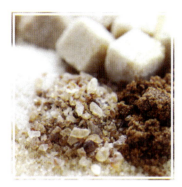

Coming off of a junk-food diet and having trouble keeping those sugar cravings in check? The glycine in gelatin can help.

On one level, glycine helps beat sugar cravings because it regulates your blood sugar levels as explained above. When your blood sugar doesn't go crashing down, your body won't feel cravings for super sugary foods to replace the glucose.

Glycine can also help you beat sugar cravings because it is very calming. It is one of the two inhibitory neurotransmitters in the body (the other is Gamma-aminolbutyric acid).[75] It helps block stress signals from the brain so they don't reach the receptor sites. I probably don't have to tell you that you will find it easier to resist sugar cravings if you aren't feeling stressed! Stress causes a flood of the hormone cortisol, which in turn causes sugar cravings because the body thinks it needs energy to deal with the stressor. Researchers at the University of Michigan found that increased stress hormones could cause sugar craving to increase by as much as three times![76]

Every single time I'm stressed and/or haven't had adequate sleep, without fail, my sugar cravings rear their ugly heads. Instead of reaching for sugary junk food, I know to grab a cup of soothing bone broth or a tasty gelatin treat instead.

GELATIN REDUCES APPETITE

Research has shown that foods high in protein can help you eat less—and gelatin is a protein. There is even evidence that gelatin might be superior to other proteins in this sense. One study showed a breakfast that contained gelatin as a protein source reduced food intake at lunch by 20% compared to other proteins.[77] However, the problem with this study is that they used gelatin by itself. Gelatin is an incomplete protein, meaning it does not contain all of the amino acids that are essential to your body. Thus, you could never use gelatin as your sole protein source in a long-term diet. But, it certainly won't hurt to add more gelatin to your life.

GELATIN BOOSTS MUSCLE FORMATION

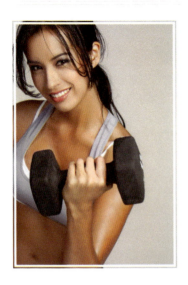

When we say that we want to lose weight, we usually mean that we want to lose *fat*. But most weight-loss diets which mainly focus on the concept of *calories in vs. calories out* don't cause fat loss. They cause you to lose *muscle mass*. Why? Because when your body is deprived of calories, it goes into "starvation mode". Your body starts breaking down the easiest form of stored energy. Unfortunately, this isn't fat. It is a heck of a lot easier for your body to break down muscle than fat, so you lose muscle weight.[78]

There are some obvious downsides to burning muscle over fat — like you will never get that sexy lean physique that you want. But the effects are probably worse than you realized *because muscle is crucial for metabolism*.

What does muscle have to do with metabolism? You've probably heard the phrase "muscle burns more calories than fat". Here is how it works:

If you've ever used one of those calorie calculator things, then you know that they always ask your current weight. This is because (putting it simply), the more body mass you have, the more calories you need to sustain yourself. So, a person who weighs 200 pounds is going to need a lot more calories daily than a person who weighs 100 pounds.

When you first begin a diet, you probably lose weight really quickly. Then, as you keep it up, the weight loss reaches a plateau. This is because you have less body mass and thus your body doesn't need as many calories daily.[79]

With this in mind, the real key to permanent weight loss is to *burn off fat while increasing (or at least maintaining) body mass*. So, it isn't going to be enough to do aerobic exercises which burn fat. You'll also need to do some anaerobic exercises which build muscle.

Consuming gelatin is by no means some magic bullet which will convert your fat into sexy lean muscle mass. However, it is a protein and protein is obviously important for when you want to build muscle. Glycine has also shown to enhance muscle repair and growth because it boosts creatine levels. It also helps regulate Human Growth Hormone (HGH) levels — you know, that hormone which people pay a fortune to have injected into their bodies and is forbidden by athlete associations because it is such a performance booster.[68] So, skip the expensive injections and opt for some gelatin instead.

Gelatin for the Brain

You know how I said earlier that diet alone isn't going to cure all of your problems—you've also got to get enough sleep and manage stress? Well, it turns out that gelatin can even help with this. The research shows that the glycine in gelatin has a calming effect on our nerves which can promote sleep and reduce stress. Okay, gelatin isn't a magic bullet that will turn you into a zen goddess, but, in combination with meditation and stress relief, here are some of the things gelatin can do for you.

GELATIN CALMS THE BODY

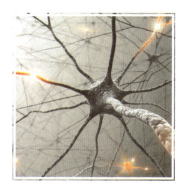

Our brains are the master control station of our nervous system. To control the nervous system, chemicals called neurotransmitters send signals throughout the body. These neurotransmitters can be excitatory or inhibitory. Excitatory neurotransmitters give us energy and focus. The inhibitory neurotransmitters calm us down. When these neurotransmitters become unbalanced, you end up feeling anxious, moody, and fatigued. You find it hard to control your appetite, have low libido, can't focus, and have trouble sleeping. There are a lot of reasons that your neurotransmitters may become imbalanced, with one of the main ones being diet.[80]

The amino acid glycine is one of the two main calming neurotransmitters in the body (the other is GABA). In the brain, it inhibits the excitatory neurotransmitters which a lot of us have in abundance due to too much stress. Glycine also gets converted into the neurotransmitter serine, which helps with focus, memory, and stress reduction.[68]

If you are having trouble sleeping, try drinking some bone broth or taking gelatin before bed. Research shows that this can help induce sleep and improve sleep quality. Gelatin will also help you get rid of daytime sleepiness.[45]

GELATIN FOR BALANCING CORTISOL LEVELS

Cortisol is the hormone which is associated with our "fight or flight" response to stress. It is actually very useful because it gives us the bursts of energy we need to deal with stressful situations. But, as you probably know by now, constant exposure to stress can have dramatic consequences for your body. Having chronic high levels of cortisol is linked to everything from weight gain to mental disorders to muscle pain.[81]

Over time, the prolonged stress can lead to adrenal fatigue in which your adrenal glands can no longer keep up with the demands of stress. You end up feeling constantly tired, get sick easily, and crave sugary foods.[82] Gelatin can help because it balances your amino acid levels, which in turn balances cortisol levels.

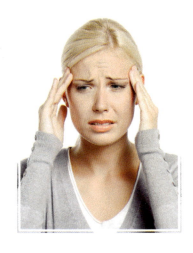

Gelatin contains the amino acid glycine which is lacking in muscle meats. In the past, humans made use of all parts of an animal, such as by making fish head soup, bone broths, and "head cheeses". Today, these parts of the animal are usually getting discarded and we just consume the muscle meats. Yes, muscle meats have a lot of important nutrients—but eating only muscle meats can cause a deficiency in glycine and an imbalance of other amino acids. This can then lead to overproduction of cortisol.

Muscle meats are high in tryptophan (that thing in turkey which is known for inducing a post-Thanksgiving coma) and cysteine. These amino acids inhibit thyroid function and mitochondrial energy production. In layman's terms, this means that the amino acids limit our ability to withstand stress. As Doctor Ray Peat explains,

"When only the muscle meats are eaten, the amino acid balance entering our blood stream is the same as that produced by extreme stress, when cortisol excess causes our muscles to be broken down to provide energy and material for repair. The formation of serotonin is increased by the excess tryptophan in muscle, and serotonin stimulates the formation of more cortisol, while the tryptophan itself, along with the excess muscle-derived cysteine, suppresses the thyroid function."[6]

Gelatin contains absolutely no tryptophan and very low levels of any of the excitatory amino acids. This is why gelatin is such an important component of a real foods diet which is rich in protein and healthy fats but low-carb (compared to the SAD diet). Switching to a real-foods diet from the SAD diet is certainly an improvement, but without the addition of glycine-rich foods like gelatin, your amino acid levels still won't be balanced. Along with gelatin, these foods are great sources of glycine:

* Kidney
* Heart
* Liver
* Spleen
* Tongue
* Tripe (stomach)
* Rinds
* Chitterlings[68]

You'll notice that these are a lot of the foods which we consider "weird" and usually discard. This goes back to what I was saying on page 24 about eating nose-to-tail. It isn't just *ethical*, it is also the way that our bodies were made to eat and healthy for us.

If you are feeling constantly tired and think that stress is to blame, then skip the coffee in the morning (this will just worsen the stress on your body). Why not drink a nice mug of bone broth instead to start your day?

GELATIN AND MOOD

As we talked about in the Gelatin for Weight Loss section, gelatin is proven to be very effective in helping to regulate blood sugar levels through gluconeogenesis. Maybe you've heard the term "Hangry" which is the half-joking term we use to describe hungry+angry. It is no surprise that hunger can affect your mood, but there is actually a neurological reason for it.

When your blood sugar levels drop, the "hunger hormone" ghrelin gets released to stimulate your appetite. Well, ghrelin also blocks serotonin, which is your "happy neurotransmitter". Okay, this is a big simplification because serotonin is involved in numerous incredibly complex neurological pathways. But, it is the neurotransmitter most linked with your mood, including depression and aggression.[83]

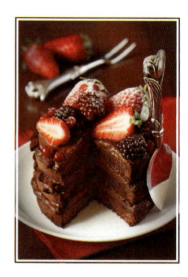

When you eat starchy or sugary foods, your serotonin levels rise again. This is a big part of the reason we find eating junk food so comforting. But those same starchy, sugary foods also make your blood sugar rise and then crash. So, you end up on a rollercoaster of serotonin highs and lows. By consuming gelatin to keep your blood sugar levels in check, you also help keep your serotonin levels in check. Yes, you can get off the rollercoaster!

By the way, about 80% of your serotonin is in the gut![84] It just goes to show that everything goes back to the gut—and we already went over the wonders that gelatin can do for your gut!

There is a reason they call your gut the "second brain" after all. You might be surprised to find out that even neurological diagnoses are often closely related to gut pathogens. I strongly recommend you check out the *Gut and Psychology Syndrome* book which is listed in the resource page to find out more about how your gut affects your overall health and what you can do about it.

Gelatin for Skin Health and Beauty

Before we get into all of the things you can do to make yourself look sexy and amazing, I want to stress that **you've got to love your body, no matter what condition it is in.**

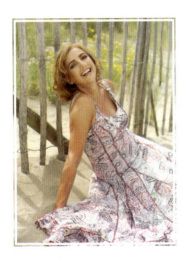

Good nutrition is one way to love our bodies, but too many people use nutrition solely as a way to get their body into a condition which they think they will be capable of loving. I realized this somewhere along my own weight loss journey. I'd always just worn hand-me-downs and frumpy clothes because I told myself that I'd buy a new wardrobe "once I lost the weight." Even when I *did* lose weight, I still didn't buy any new clothes. I hid under awful baggy clothing and didn't bother taking any "before" and "after" pictures. Why? Because I didn't consider myself "finished". Even though I was looking (and feeling) so much better, I still couldn't allow myself to be happy with my body. This negative self image was holding me back from enjoying life.

It took a long time before I allowed myself to fully enjoy my new body. Once I did, the transformation was outstanding. It wasn't just my new figure and glowing skin which was getting me complements. It was the fact that I was exuding confidence. What am I trying to say? Well, for starters, there are a lot of ways to love our bodies. Nutrition, exercise, and pampering are just some. I'm not saying that striving to lose weight or improve your skin is a bad thing. But obsessing over it and holding unrealistic photoshopped models as the ideal is one of the worst things we can do. Don't hold yourself back from enjoying life until you meet certain goals. It simply isn't healthy and it certainly isn't any fun!

As for nutrition and beauty, I find it ironic that as a society we spend so much on beauty products and will even torture ourselves with "treatments" like Botox in which we inject toxins into our faces just to temporarily tighten the skin (this is definitely *not* my idea of loving your body!). It is ironic because people will go through all these torturous treatments, but balk at the idea of changing their diets. Yet, diet is one of the most important factors to looking great.

If you are deficient in nutrients, it is only logical that this will show in the health of your skin, hair, nails, and teeth. Having skin issues or poor dental health is really just a canary in the coal mine letting us know something is wrong. If you haven't already, the gut section of this eBook is a must read as that is the hub to the rest of our body and the imperative starting point for healing. Gelatin, by giving you a dosage of collagen, is one of the best beauty superfoods you can consume.

GELATIN FOR SKIN HEALTH

Your skin isn't just an organ; it is actually the largest organ of the human body. The skin is part of the immune system. This might sound weird at first, but then consider the fact that your skin is one of the only organs which actually comes into contact with the real world. It blocks pathogens, toxins, and other harmful substances from entering the body. It also helps get harmful substances out of the body, such as by secreting them from the pores. While skin might be part of the immune system, it is your gut which is in charge of the immune system. If your gut isn't working properly, then your immune system can't function well either.[85]

Healing Your Gut to Treat Skin Problems

There is no shortage of studies which show the link between gut health and skin health. One study found that 40% of people with acne also had low stomach acid. Another study found that adolescents with acne were more likely to have bloating.[86] A Russian study found that more than half of people with acne problems also had altered gut flora. Another study found that probiotics can help cure acne.[87] And the list of evidence goes on...

The gut can also be linked to just about every type of skin breakout or rash. It may seem weird that your gut health would affect your skin. But then consider the fact that your skin is teeming with bacteria. There are about 1 million bacteria living on *each square centimeter* of your skin. Overall, the bacteria in our entire body outnumber human cells 10 to 1.[88]

As we talked about earlier in the gut health section, gelatin is very good for gut health. It stimulates stomach acid production, which is important for healthy gut bacteria to thrive. In this sense, gelatin can do wonders for treating skin conditions like acne. Even skin conditions like psoriasis and eczema, which are considered autoimmune conditions, can be treated with gelatin because of the connection between leaky gut and autoimmunity. Another way gelatin helps get rid of acne and skin problems is by assisting the liver in flushing out toxins so they don't manifest in the skin.[86,89]

Gelatin Can Help with Hormonal Acne Too

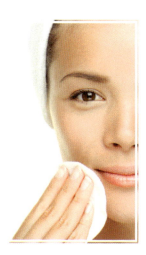

Not all acne is directly linked to digestive health. If your acne is occurring around the mouth or jawline, it is likely hormonal instead of gut-related. For females, another big sign that your acne is hormonal is that breakouts primarily occur during certain times of your menstrual cycle.[90]

Gelatin can help control this hormonal acne in a number of ways. First off, the glycine in gelatin is also considered an antiestrogenic substance, which can help balance hormones and reduce breakouts.[6] Gelatin also helps alleviate stress (which we talk about in the Gelatin for the Brain section) and acts as an anti-inflammatory. Stress doesn't directly cause acne, but it can create bodily conditions conducive to acne (like upsetting the digestive system). Stress also causes inflammation, which worsens acne. As an anti-inflammatory substance, gelatin can also reduce inflammation to the pores.[90]

Of course, you'll have to do more than just supplement with gelatin if you want great-looking skin. You'll also have to avoid foods which are bad for gut health (like processed sugars and grains) and balance your gut flora by consuming probiotics (such as the delicious Kombucha Jello or quality sauerkraut or pickles such as those listed on the resource page). But gelatin can be an important component of your overall skin health. Gelatin-rich bone broth can do even more wonders for your skin because it contains many components which directly benefit the skin, like hyaluronic acid which keeps skin moist and keratin which protects the skin from harmful substances.[91]

GELATIN FOR WRINKLES

Collagen is what gives our skin its elasticity. When collagen in the skin starts to break down, the skin becomes thinner and creases (aka wrinkles) form. Sure, there are all sorts of dangerous solutions like Botox available. But, if you want longer lasting (and safer) results, you've got to increase your collagen levels.

You can apply collagen creams to your face to get rid of wrinkles, but the skin can't absorb collagen because the molecules are too big.[14] There is also the possibility of injecting collagen into your face to replace lost collagen. This is actually pretty effective (though expensive, painful, and fairly risky). But, even this isn't a permanent solution because your body will break down that collagen so you'll have to go in for another injection.[92]

That leaves us with oral collagen supplements. You could take pills that cost over $1000 for a few doses, but why not stick with gelatin which is much more affordable and something you can even get the kids to eat as well? Gelatin has shown to have a very high bioavailability (meaning your body absorbs it well) and even the quality brands like those recommended in the resource page) are really affordable. If you make bone broth to get gelatin, then it is only going to cost you a few cents.

Studies show that collagen peptides from gelatin are easily absorbed by the body and make their way to where they are needed.[33, 34] This helps reduce collagen breakdown, reducing the quantity of wrinkles! Since consuming gelatin has shown to rebuild lost collagen in joints, we could also assume that gelatin might be able to *reverse wrinkles* by rebuilding lost skin collagen. There are a few studies which do show that collagen can reverse wrinkles but, unfortunately, most of these studies only focus on a specific collagen peptide so we can't be sure about the exact benefits of gelatin for reversing wrinkles.

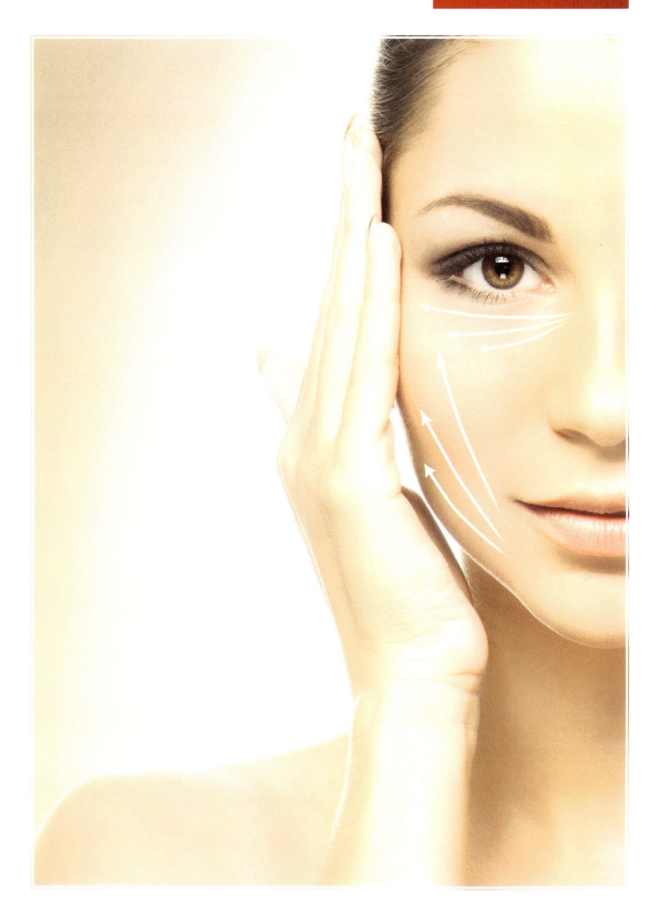

HOLLYWOOD HOMESTEAD

The Gelatin Secret   67

GELATIN FOR CELLULITE

Cellulite has become a national obsession lately. Why? Probably because 80–90% of women have it![93] Since nearly everyone has cellulite to some degree, you'd think that people would accept it by now. No. That isn't what our culture does. It instead stigmatizes it by calling it a "flaw" and makes you feel ashamed for having something which is completely normal. Then they try to sell you all sorts of "treatments." What I'm saying is cellulite is *normal*. Athletes have cellulite. Skinny people have cellulite. Celebrities have cellulite. People who undergo plastic surgery have cellulite…

I really hope that you aren't going to start chugging bone broth only because of what I am about to say about gelatin and cellulite. You *should* chug it because you love your body enough to take care of it! With that said, gelatin can have the extra benefit of preventing or reducing cellulite.

Cellulite is caused by a combination of two factors: fat and collagen. When our skin is healthy and contains adequate amounts of collagen, it creates a smooth covering over our bodies. If collagen becomes weak or develops holes in it though, then the fat underneath our skin will poke through and make those lumps we call cellulite. Reducing your body fat may help cellulite but, since we all still need some fat on our bodies, you also have to boost collagen if you want to get rid of cellulite.[94] As we talked about earlier, gelatin is a good source of collagen that your body can absorb and use.

While we are at it, gelatin can also help you shed the fat off of your body. Ever wonder why women get collagen more often than men? It is because our female bodies are made very differently. We all have alpha receptions (which produce fat cells) and beta receptors (which break down fat). Sorry to break the news ladies, but we've got about *9x* more fat-producing cells in our hips and thighs than men! This is also the same area where most of our estrogen receptors are—and women also have more estrogen than men. As you may remember, estrogen *makes* fat cells whereas testosterone breaks them down.[95]

In older women, lower levels of estrogen can contribute to the breakdown of collagen. Interestingly, just the opposite occurs in younger women. If there is too much estrogen, collagen can also break down. Because of poor diet, stress, lack of exercise, and consumption of phytoestrogen foods like soy, many young women these days are experiencing a condition called *estrogen dominance*. This is something that can be diagnosed and treated with supplements under the guidance of a naturopathic doctor.

The glycine in gelatin has shown to act as an anti-estrogenic substance[6], which means that it can balance your hormones so you break down those globs of fat which are causing cellulite while also keeping/rebuilding your collagen. Reducing estrogen dominance can also solve problems like varicose veins, fibroids in the uterus, cervical dysplasia, endometriosis, ovarian cysts, and gallstones.[95] We'll get more into gelatin and estrogen dominance in the next chapter.

GELATIN FOR HAIR

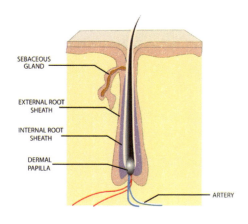

HAIR STRUCTURE

Your hair might be made from dead cells, but it is important to remember that those cells were once *alive*. And, like all living cells, hair needs good nutrition if it is going to be healthy.

Hair growth starts inside follicles that are within the skin. Follicles are basically a sheath of collagen which holds and nurtures the hair from the root. At the very base of the follicle is something called the *papilla* which is also made from collagen. It is what links the follicle to the rest of the body. The *hair bulb* is situated directly above the papilla. The papilla provides the hair bulb with nutrients in order to create new hair cells. As the hair cells are pushed upwards, they go through a process called keratinization. The hair cells are filled with fibrous proteins and lose their nucleus (which is why we say hair is dead). As the dead hair cells stack up, the hair is pushed out of the follicle and our hair "grows." The hair that exits the skin is just a strand of woven keratin proteins—about 91% protein to be exact. Depending on genetic components, hair cell proteins can form in different ways, resulting in different textures of hair.[96, 97, 98]

You will notice that the hair follicle and the papilla are both made up of collagen. So, it should go without saying that consuming collagen is important for your hair health. Just like how collagen keeps your skin looking supple, it also helps each strand of hair maintain its strength and thickness. The healthier your hair follicles are, the larger they will be and will produce healthier, stronger hair.[97, 99]

If you want lush, thick hair, then consuming gelatin is going to help a heck of a lot more than any of those expensive hair treatments you find at a salon. Okay, it does take a while before you start noticing any improvement, especially since hair takes so long to grow out and you'll still have a sheath of unhealthy hair hanging off of you. If you want a quick way to make your hair look great, you can simply apply some gelatin.

Here is one solution you can use when you feel like your hair needs some extra conditioning.

Mix 1 Tbsp of gelatin powder (*don't use collagen hydrolysate because it won't gel!) with ½ cup of cool water. Then add another ½ cup of warm water plus 1 tsp of apple cider vinegar and a teaspoon of honey. It forms a nice gel that you can apply to your hair. Leave on for at least 5 minutes. If your hair is really dry and lackluster, you might need to do this 3 times a week for starters.

The reason that the gelatin treatment for hair works so well is because gelatin is a protein (remember, your hair is 91% protein). Collagen also remarkably resembles keratin in that they are both types of fibrous proteins. They even share some of the same amino acids.[100]

You can try all you want to fix your hair problems from the outside, but it probably isn't going to do you much good. Heck, a lot of those so-called solutions are actually making the problem worse. Take conventional shampoo. Typical ingredients in shampoo include parabens (which are skin irritants and cause hormone disruptions), alcohol (which is incredibly drying) and Sodium laurel sulfate (which is used to make shampoo foam but destroys hair follicles). Plus, these shampoos are so strong that they strip your hair of all of the natural oils it needs to stay moisturized. Considering all of this, no wonder you've got dry brittle hair and dandruff![101]

So what are you supposed to use to clean your hair if conventional products are off limits? One option is to spring for those expensive gourmet all-natural brands of shampoo that are free of parabens and SLS. Or you can just make your own natural hair care solutions. Yes, I know it sounds scary to ditch the shampoo and you worry you might be labeled a hippy. But you'd be surprised how great your hair will look.

For cleaning your hair, a mixture of 2 Tbsp baking soda dissolved into 1 cup of warm water does the trick. For conditioning, mix 2 Tbsp of unfiltered apple cider vinegar in 1 cup of warm water, plus a few drops of lavender oil. To get the lowdown on natural hair care, you'll want to read *Skintervention* by Liz Wolfe, which you can find on the resource page. The solutions recommended in the book aren't just effective, they are also super easy.

Note: you can also make your own hair gel out of gelatin! Just mix ¼ tsp gelatin with ½ cup hot water. Let it set and add essential oils if you want. Now you're ready to go! Just remember to keep it stored in the refrigerator and it will last about 2 weeks.

GELATIN FOR NAILS

Just like hair, our nails are made from keratin. The reason that nails are harder than hair is because they contain different amino acid profiles. Some say that you can strengthen your fingernails by soaking them in gelatin. The idea is that, because gelatin is a protein just like keratin is a protein, that the gelatin will strengthen them. True, some of the proteins in gelatin might be absorbed into the nails — but the effectiveness of this is really debatable. Plus, we know that if you want to have healthy-looking fingers and nails, it all starts with internal health and healthy nutrient levels.

Unlike with hair, our nails do *not* grow out of a sheath of collagen. So, consuming gelatin isn't going to directly help your nails be healthier. To get healthy nails, you need to focus on getting enough of certain nutrients, including:

* **Zinc**: Inadequate zinc leads to brittle nails; white spots on nails is a sign of zinc deficiency

* **Biotin**: Biotin deficiency leads to brittle, weak nails

* **Iron**: Inadequate iron will cause nails to become brittle and also get a spoon shape in which they curve in the middle[102]

Gelatin doesn't contain any of these nutrients, but it does help with our gut health which is ESSENTIAL to absorbing nutrients. In other words, you can pop supplements all day long and even eat amazing nutrient dense food but, if your gut is damaged, your intestines are essentially going to be on strike and prevent you from absorbing a lot of those nutrients. I guess you could get around this problem by giving yourself expensive intramuscular vitamin injections. But that would only be a short-term Band-Aid. Why not focus instead on healing your gut with the help of grass fed gelatin?[85]

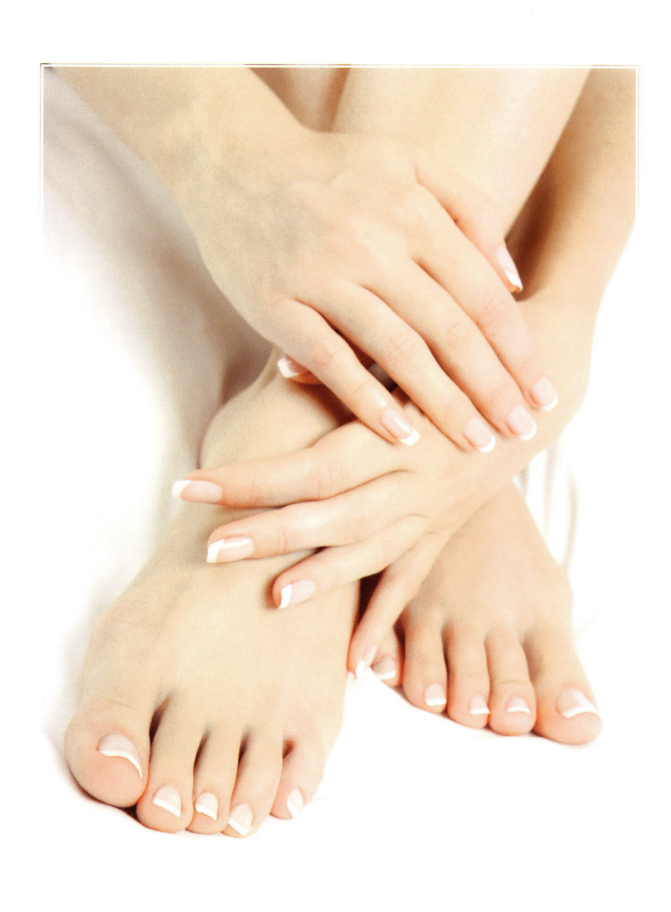

SUPER SIMPLE SKIN CARE ROUTINE

My cabinets used to be filled with all sorts of "beauty products" which were supposedly going to get rid of acne, reduce wrinkles, tone my skin, moisturize it, and you name it. I wouldn't have believed you then if you'd told me I'd be ditching all of these expensive products for simple DIY options, and that the DIY solutions would be more effective — not to mention a whole heck of a lot cheaper!

For anyone who wants better looking skin (who doesn't?), I recommend *The Skintervention Guide* by Liz Wolfe. It is basically the bible of skincare and talks all about how to fix your skin from the inside out. You can find it on the resource page.

Here is what my skincare routine looks like right now. This is a basic cleansing routine that would work for any skin type. Of course you can personalize it based on your needs and the recommendations in the *Skintervention Guide*. Preferably, you should only cleanse once a day in the evening:

- **Oil cleansing**: Simply rub a thin layer of coconut or jojoba oil on your face massaging gently. With a warm washcloth wipe it off.

- **Toning**: With a cotton ball or washcloth gently wipe a solution of 5 parts filtered water, 1 part organic raw unfiltered apple cider vinegar on your face.

- **Moisturizing**: use a dab of the same oil (coconut or jojoba) to apply a very thin layer on your face as a moisturizer.

With skin care, remember that less is usually more. By less, I mean less scrubbing and cleansing and less ingredients. Real beauty starts from the inside out, so getting yourself healthy is going to do a lot more than any of those expensive beauty treatments could!

Gelatin for Dental Health

As we talked about in the bone health section, gelatin can do wonders for your bones. Since both bones and teeth are hard, white, and composed of calcium and other minerals, one might assume that gelatin acts on them in the same way. But, really, bones and teeth are very different substances.

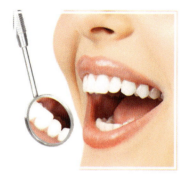

Bones are mostly made out of collagen which is studded with minerals like calcium, phosphorus, and sodium. Since collagen is a living tissue, it can regenerate itself. Bones also contain osteoblast cells which are in charge of forming new bone tissue.

By contrast, teeth do not contain much collagen. In fact, the outer part of teeth (enamel) does not contain any collagen. Instead, it is made out of large amounts of minerals. This makes sense, right? After all, collagen is a soft substance, and we need our teeth to be very hard in order to tear through food. Our teeth are actually the hardest part of our body.[103] Because enamel does not contain collagen or osteoblast cells, it does not repair itself like bone does. However, this does *not* mean that your teeth can't be healed or nourished! Let's explore this idea a bit further…

ANATOMY OF THE TEETH

Before we get into the details of how gelatin and healthy diet can help you fight and reverse tooth decay, we'll need to go over the parts of the teeth. Basically, teeth are made up of four layers. From the outermost inwards, they are:

- **Enamel**: This is the hard, shiny coating of your teeth. It is made up of about 96% minerals.

- **Dentin**: Dentin is located underneath enamel. It goes down into our gums and surrounds the outer part of the tooth root. It is mostly made up of minerals but also contains collagen. This makes it softer than enamel. If your enamel wears away, the dentin becomes exposed and is susceptible to cavities because of its softness.

- **Centenum**: The centenum covers the tooth root and gives the tooth stability by attaching to periodontal ligaments. It has a high composition of collagen.

- **Pulp**: The pulp is the central-most part of the tooth. It has a hole at its base (the root) where it connects to blood vessels and nerves. The pulp is incredibly important for tooth health because it provides nutrients to the teeth, including minerals needed for remineralizing the enamel. Tooth pulp contains collagen![104]

You will notice that most parts of the teeth (all but the enamel) contain some collagen. We will get into the significance of this when we talk about the ways to cure tooth decay. But you will note that modern dental health recommendations only talk about brushing and flossing. This does nothing but clean the enamel (and sometimes strip the teeth of its enamel and irritate the gums[105]). To really cure tooth decay, you've got to heal *all* parts of the teeth.

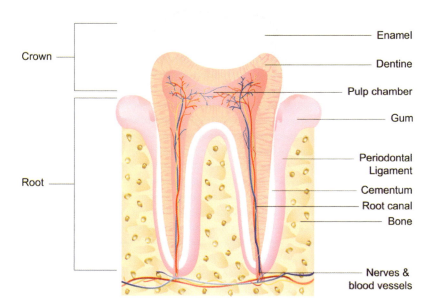

TOOTH ANATOMY

WHY BRUSHING WON'T STOP TOOTH DECAY

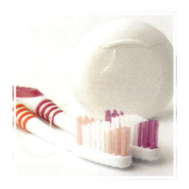

Modern dentistry blames tooth decay on bacteria which feed on the residue of sugary foods on our teeth. They say that the bacteria produce acids which break down enamel and cause cavities and tooth decay. Their solution? Avoid sugary foods and brush and floss your teeth daily.

If this recommendation were effective, we wouldn't have an epidemic of tooth decay on our hands and tooth decay wouldn't be a problem which only worsens with age. I'm not saying that modern dentistry is completely incorrect in saying that sugary food causes tooth decay. Bacteria does feed on sugar residues in the mouth, forming acid which wears away the teeth. This was first hypothesized by a dentist named W. D. Miller who found that teeth put into a mixture of fermenting bread and saliva would erode. Interestingly, Miller believed that strong teeth would not decay, even in the presence of acids. He said,

"The extent to which any tooth suffers from the action of the acid depends upon its density and structure, but more particularly upon the perfection of the enamel and the protection of the neck of the tooth by healthy gums. What we might call the perfect tooth would resist indefinitely the same acid to which a tooth of opposite character would succumb in a few weeks."[105]

Aside from the bacterial aspect of tooth decay, refined sugar can wreak havoc on your teeth in other ways. It causes hormonal imbalances which impact calcium absorption, alter the acidity of your saliva, and inflame your gums. Though modern dentistry insists that the problem and solution are external (bacteria and brushing), the real problem and solution come from within.

A healthy tooth contains about 3 *miles* of tubes (that's per tooth!) that are filled with a fluid similar to that found in the spinal cord. Tooth enamel also contains small amounts (about 2%) of this fluid. These tubes are the growing parts of a tooth. They feed the dentin and enamel with odontoblast cells, which are like mini pumps. The odontoblasts feed nutrients to the tooth and remove corrosive materials. As Ramiel Nagel points out in *Cure Tooth Decay*, a healthy tooth basically cleans itself out. He redefines tooth decay as a combination of odontoporosis (decreased tooth density) and odontoclasia (the absorption and destruction of tooth tissue).[105]

WESTON A. PRICE LINKS TOOTH DECAY TO DIET

Almost 100 years ago, a visionary dentist by the name of Weston Price realized something was wrong. When he looked into his patients' mouths, he mostly found rampant tooth decay. This was usually accompanied by a myriad of other health problems, like arthritis, diabetes, and chronic fatigue. Unlike many other "health experts" of the time, he did not believe that these deformities and disabilities were part of "God's plan for mankind".

Could there be a connection between tooth health and general health?

Price got the crazy idea (at least they thought it was crazy then) to travel to remote, isolated parts of the world and study the health of people who had not been touched by modern civilization.

What do you think he found?

His research led to the publication of *Nutrition and Physical Degeneration* in 1939. Interestingly, these "primitive" people often had perfectly straight, white teeth. It wasn't just genetics either. In people who had come into contact with missionaries and had abandoned their traditional diets, their perfect teeth then began to resemble those of people in civilized cultures: rampant with decay.[106]

As a result of his research, Price concluded that dental health was determined by diet. In particular he found that these 3 aspects were vital for dental health:

* Having enough minerals in the diet

* Having enough fat-soluble vitamins in the diet (like vitamins A, D, E, and K)

* How readily the body is absorbing those vitamins and minerals (which we talk lots about in the gut section of this book)

Of course, there are other issues which can contribute to tooth decay, like hormonal imbalances and excess consumption of things like coffee. But, these 3 identified by Dr. Price are the big ones.

I highly recommend you read Dr. Price's book (you can find it on the resource page). It is surprisingly not outdated and is an interesting read for anyone who wants to learn more about the origins of the real food movement.

HOW TO CURE TOOTH DECAY WITH DIET

If you want to cure tooth decay, you have to address each of the dietary issues identified by Dr. Price: inadequate minerals in the diet, inadequate fat-soluble vitamins in the diet, and poor absorption of dietary nutrients. Gelatin isn't going to be a cure-all, but it can help. Remember that, as we discussed in the gut section, without a healthy gut, which gelatin can help you repair, you likely will not absorb a lot of the nutrients you are consuming. Just because they are going in your mouth does not mean they are getting distributed throughout your body!

Getting Enough Minerals in the Diet

Tooth enamel has the highest concentration of minerals in the entire body. Along with calcium, deficiencies in the minerals iron, magnesium, copper, manganese, and phosphorus are linked with tooth decay[105,107] While gelatin alone might not have these minerals, bone broth is a great source of them (and many other nutrients as well). This is why Dr. Price's original protocol for treating tooth decay included almost-daily ingestion of bone broth, which is impossible to overdose on. According to the fantastic book *Cure Tooth Decay* by Ramiel Nagel, fish broth is the best broth for curing tooth decay. It should be made from wild fish and include the carcass, head, and organs.[105]

Now, it is always best to get these minerals through food. But, if you want to directly give your teeth some minerals they can use to heal themselves, then you might want to consider using a remineralizing toothpaste. The toothpaste, which is really easy to make yourself, contains minerals for nourishing your teeth. It can also help draw toxins out of your teeth.

SQUEEZABLE REMINERALIZING TOOTHPASTE RECIPE

Ingredients:

- 3 Tbsp calcium powder
- 3 Tbsp coconut oil
- 3 Tbsp xylitol
- 2 Tbsp filtered water
- 2 tsp baking soda
- 1 tsp bentonite clay
- ½ tsp calcium/magnesium powder
- 40 drops peppermint essential oils
- 20 drops trace minerals

(see the resource page for where to buy these ingredients)

Directions:

1. Mix thoroughly with a spoon (you may need to heat the coconut oil a bit to do this).
2. Store in your squeezable bottle. (Piping it in with a plastic bag was very helpful).
3. Brush twice a day!

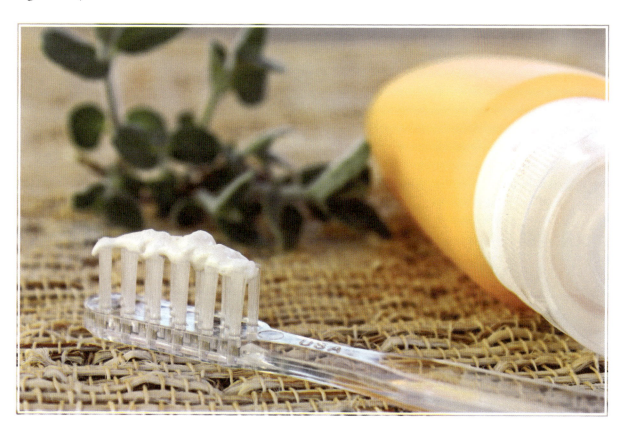

Getting Enough Fat-Soluble Vitamins in the Diet

What does fat have to do with your teeth? Fat-soluble vitamins are vital for helping the body absorb minerals. You probably already know about vitamin D's role in absorbing calcium, but you might not know about the importance of the other fat-soluble vitamins though and their various benefits.

- **Vitamin A**: Needed for bone growth, tissue repair, and protecting the body from toxins

- **Vitamin D**: Helps the body absorb calcium and phosphorus (both important teeth minerals)

- **Vitamin E**: Is an antioxidant which helps with tissue healing and circulation

- **Vitamin K2**: Transports calcium to where it is needed in the body[105]

As a child, I had horrendous teeth. I didn't consume many sweets and I religiously brushed my teeth twice a day. My mother was very health conscious and I only managed to get my hands on a soda about once a month. So, why did I always have multiple cavities every time I went to the dentist?

I attribute my poor dental health to the fact that I was eating a very low fat vegetarian diet which was devoid of just about all the fat soluble vitamins needed for good dental health. Coupled with all the high phytate-containing foods I was eating almost exclusively like grains and soy, it is no wonder that I was a dental disaster!

Now, I eat a real foods diet which is rich in fat-soluble vitamins. I also largely credit fermented cod liver oil (FCLO) for helping me restore my dental health). Fermented cod liver oil is incredibly rich in fat-soluble vitamins. Just a single teaspoon of the oil has the same amount of vitamin D as 18 ounces of salmon or 5 dozen eggs. A teaspoon also has as much vitamin A as 2 gallons of milk or 2 ounces of chicken liver.[107] Another instrumental supplement for me has been high-vitamin butter oil. I buy a blend which has both fermented cod liver oil and butter oil. You can find it on the [resource page](). It differs from regular butter in that it is made from the butter fat of grass-fed cows by putting it into a centrifuge to produce a nutrient-dense oil. It is incredibly rich in vitamin K2.[107]

Honestly, in the beginning of my tooth-healing journey, when I ran out of my FCLO/butter oil blend for a couple weeks, I could feel my tooth sensitivity returning. For good measure I still take it today as does the rest of my family.

Absorbing Tooth Vitamins and Minerals

You can take supplements all you want but, if your body isn't absorbing them properly, then you aren't going to help your teeth. As we talked about in the Gelatin for Gut Health section, gelatin can help this problem because it heals the gut. However, gelatin might be able to help the teeth absorb more nutrients in an even more direct way.

You'll remember that the inner parts of the teeth all contain some collagen. These parts are responsible for delivering nutrients to your teeth, including minerals to the enamel. By supplement with gelatin, you provide your teeth with a good source of dietary collagen that your body can readily absorb.

As Adele Boskey discusses in her article about the mineralization of bone and teeth, "collagen provides the template for mineral deposition in dentin and bone, and the size and organization of the collagen fibrils limits the dimensions that mineral crystals can attain." So, by improving the health of your inner tooth, you are making it possible for the tooth to receive the minerals it needs to prevent decay.[108] Since collagen is the connective tissue which actually anchors your teeth in place, it is also incredibly important for preventing tooth loss. In particular, a part of collagen known as *glycosaminoglycans* (GAGS) have shown to repair compromised gum tissue.[109]

While you are at it, you will also need to avoid substances which draw minerals out of your body. Phytates (phytic acid) like those found in grains, beans, soy, and nuts are big culprits.[105] I would encourage largely avoiding them regardless, but it is especially important to at least avoid them during your tooth remineralization phase.

TOOTH HEALING IS POSSIBLE

The fact that I suffered from poor diet during my formative years is something that will likely take me a lifetime to recover from as those are the years that are most crucial to building long term health. However, I am happy to say that I've already seen vast improvements since I adopted a real foods diet and lifestyle. My teeth are no longer translucent. They are solid. For the first time in my entire life, I have not gotten cavities in years. The dentist can't believe it. My gums don't feel tender when I brush and I no longer cringe with pain during a dental cleaning.

I used to joke with the dentist that he should just give me dentures and call it a day. I thought it was just my destiny to have awful teeth health for the rest of my life and I'm honestly shocked at how quickly my tooth health took a turn for the better once I cleaned up my diet and started focusing on gut health. Healing won't happen overnight but, if you make diet and lifestyle changes, you will see benefits.

I encourage you to focus on gut healing as described in the gut section of this book, such as by incorporating gelatin, healthy fats, and fat soluble vitamins into your diet.

For more information on reversing cavities and curing and preventing tooth decay, I strongly recommend the book *Cure Tooth Decay* by Ramiel Nagel.

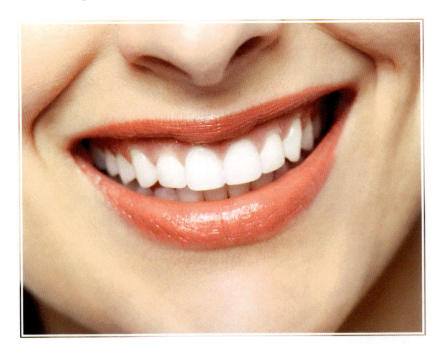

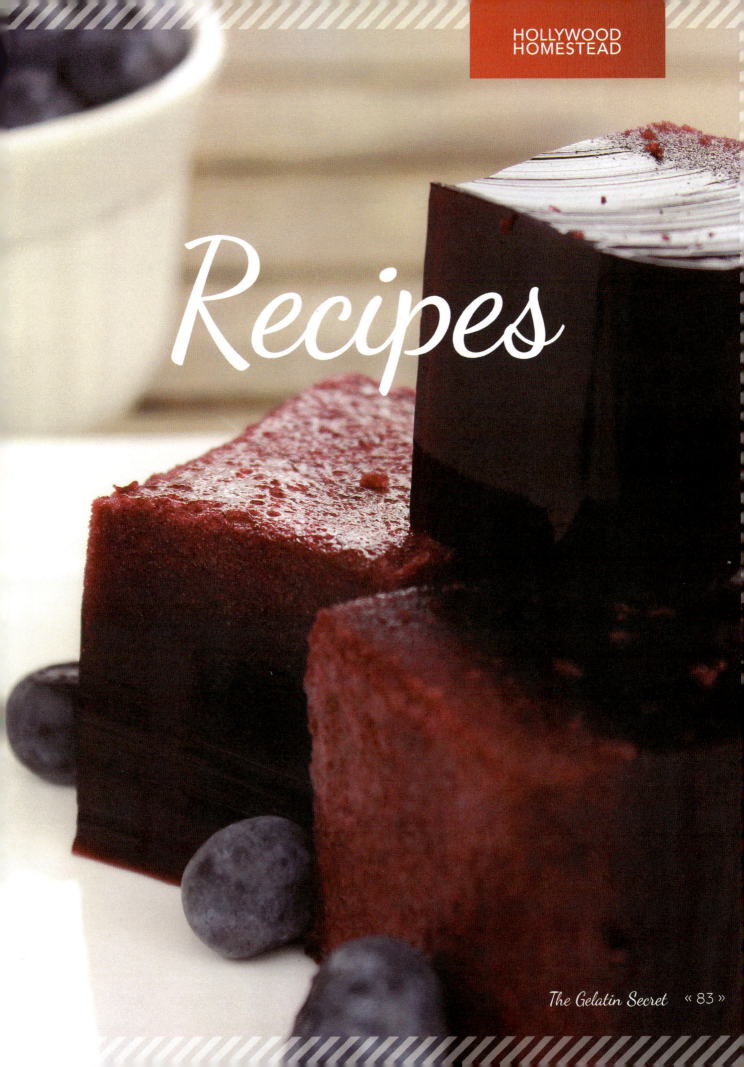
Recipes

SECTION 04

Recipes

The recipes I've included in this eBook require virtually no experience in the kitchen. They're easy to make and the ingredients are easy to source. I wanted to make it as easy as possible for you to include as much gelatin in your diet as possible.

But, this wouldn't be a book about gelatin without mentioning a couple of classic recipes like aspic and head cheese.

Fair warning, even some of my long time foodie friends are repulsed at the idea of head cheese and I have never tried to make either of these at home.

What is aspic?

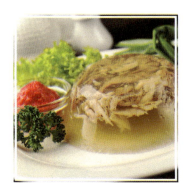

Aspic, a popular dish in the United States in the 1950s, is essentially a savory jello, made with bone broth and/or gelatin powder. There are a variety of aspic recipes out there. It is a very versatile dish in that you can include different chunks of meat, vegetables and even fruit in it! You may have heard of it referred to as a gelatin salad.

Another dish that is worth mentioning is head cheese. Now, if aspic sounded unappetizing and the picture of chicken feet in the bone broth section makes you cringe, you might want to consider skipping to the next section right about now...

What is head cheese?

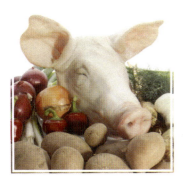

Head cheese is not cheese at all. It is made from an entire pig head which is cooked for several hours along with vegetables and spices until tender. After being chopped and thoroughly mixed to together it is placed in the refrigerator in a loaf pan to set like a jello would be. You then slice it almost like a loaf of bread. It is gelatinous and chunky and incredibly nutrient dense. If you can get past the idea of it, you'll notice it is quite delicious. My friends Sean and Suzanne made it recently and I was blown away at how tasty it was. It is by far the most nutrient dense food I've eaten all year.

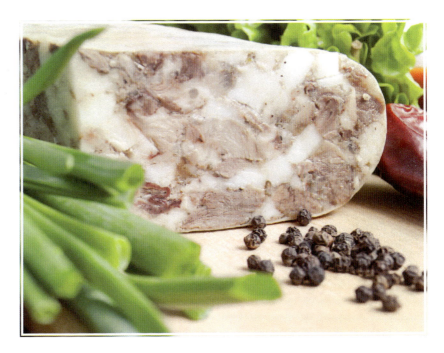

For complete instructions on how to make it please visit their blog: http://freerange-human.com/recipes/spiced-cider-brined-head-cheese/

As I mentioned earlier in this book, ever since I started eating meat a few years ago, I felt compelled to take into account the sacrifice of the animal I was consuming and move towards a more sustainable, nose-to-tail approach. Simply put, this means consuming every part of the animal. Head cheese is almost imperative when eating nose-to-tail. If you're interested in exploring this idea further, the book *Beyond Bacon* by Stacy Toth and Matthew McCarry is chock full of recipes that respect the whole hog. I also love the incredibly beautiful and useful video called *The Anatomy of Thrift* by Farmstead Meatsmith found here: http://anatomyofthrift.com/

Guide to Making Gelatin-Rich Bone Broth

Bone broth is what you perhaps know of as your grandmother's chicken stock. It is made by simply cooking down quality bones to extract the minerals and collagen into liquid form so we can consume it and absorb the goodness. The difference between broth and stock is simply that broth is usually cooked for a lot longer to extract more nutrients from the bones.

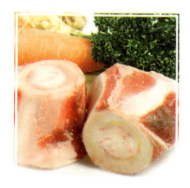

You can either drink bone broth straight up like I often do, typically a mug a day in the cold months, or add it to soups, vegetables, sauces, you name it! You can make bone broth out of any animal bones you'd like and in this section I will go over the various methods you can use to make broth. In the following sections of this eBook you'll see several ideas and recipes to get you started.

If you're new to bone broth I would definitely recommend starting with chicken broth as it is the most palatable and the one with the most pleasant aroma. I would also recommend starting with the slow cooker method, if you have one, since it is the one that is the lowest maintenance option.

A note about quality: *the quality of bones is important! Of course I would still recommend you make and consume broth regardless of the quality you can afford. However, to maximize the nutrient density of your broth, I would recommend making an effort to purchase bones from pastured or wild ruminants and poultry and wild caught fish. This is not only more ethical, but studies show that grass-fed, free-range animals also are more nutritious.*

MAKING SENSE OF BONE QUALITY

Are you confused by the labels on your meat and signs at the grocery store? I don't blame you! Here is a handy chart to use when purchasing the most common bones (and meat for that matter). Of course, wild game is also fair… game. This is just a starting point to help you better navigate the grocery store.

If you'd like to find a local farmer in your area, www.eatwild.com is a great place to start. Avoiding CAFO (Concentrated Animal Feeding Operation) meat and bones is advisable.

When it comes to ingredients, quality is important but it's also about making the best choices you can which are within your budget and available. Just do the best you can and improve when and where you can.

	BEEF AND LAMB	PORK	POULTRY	FISH
Best	Grass Fed and Finished	Pastured	Pastured	Wild Caught
Better	Grass Fed	–	Organic	–
Good	Organic	Organic	Antibiotic and Hormone Free	Sustainably (Eco) Farmed
Ok	Antibiotic Free	Antibiotic Free	Free Range and Cage Free	Farmed

I usually roast a couple of chickens each week and save the bones in a freezer bag to make broth with later. Any time we eat any meat with bones, those bones go in a freezer bag destined for broth.

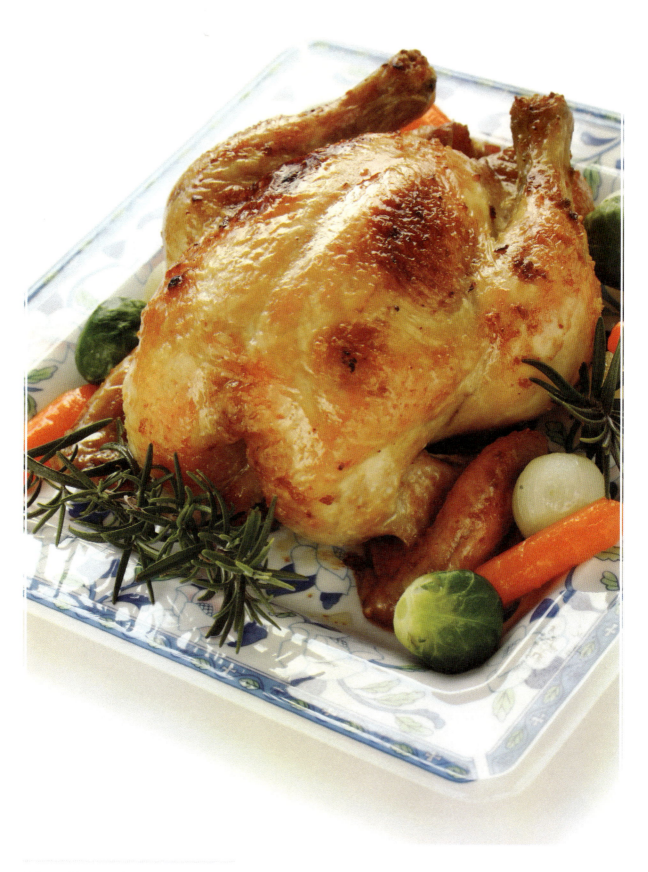

DIFFERENT TYPES OF BONE BROTH:

CHICKEN (most palatable, best for beginners)

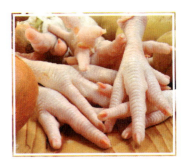

I'll admit, this is the broth I make most often, mainly because we always have chicken bones on hand from our roasted chickens and also because it is the most palatable. Since we make it in the crock pot and have a batch going almost constantly, it is the one with the most pleasant aroma as well. When I have them on hand, I like to add chicken heads and feet since they give my broth an extra boost of gelatin.

BEEF, LAMB and other ruminants (most nutritious)

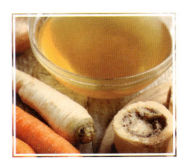

The consensus is that broth made from large ruminants like cows is the most nutritious. This is because the broth has a better ratio of Omega 3 to Omega 6 fatty acids than with broth from fowl. Also, ruminant bones are usually rich in marrow, which is full of minerals (but is also what gives this broth a less palatable taste). You'll also probably notice right away that your ruminant broths are much more gelatinous than other broths. Of course, the nutritional value of the broth depends on which bones you are using. You can use any bones but try mixing marrow bones (for the minerals) with knuckle bones (which are especially rich in collagen). For better flavor, you might consider the additional step of roasting these bones before making your broth. This will get rid of the slightly bitter taste of the marrow.[110,111,112]

FISH (fastest)

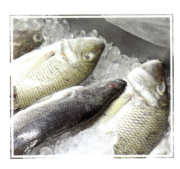

Since fish bones are the smallest, it is only logical that they are the fastest to break down. They are also very affordable. You can use the head and carcass of the fish as well. Your grocery store will likely not have heads, so you'll have to get it from your local fish market. It is best to use non-fatty fish because the oils in fatty fish could go rancid during cooking.[113] Fatty fish also make for a smelly broth! Make sure you remove the gills and eyes before you start cooking.[114]

Recommended fish are halibut, cod, flounder, sole, St. Pierre, and Rascasse. Avoid fatty fish like salmon, trout, and mackerel.[114,115]

DIFFERENT METHODS OF COOKING BONE BROTH:

Slow Cooker Method: (lowest maintenance, great for beginners)

What you will need:

- Quality bones: as little or as many as you want—2lbs is a good starting point, either frozen or thawed
- Filtered water
- 1–2 Tbsp Organic unfiltered Apple Cider Vinegar
- Slow cooker

Slow Cooker Directions:

1. Turn the slow cooker on "High"
2. Add your bones to the slow cooker. They can be frozen or thawed. The more bones you add, the thicker the broth will be. I typically add the carcasses of 2 roast chickens and some extra chicken heads and feet I get from my local farmer.
3. If you'd like, add some vegetable scraps like onions, carrots, and celery for flavor. I usually keep it pretty minimal so I can salt and flavor later as needed depending on what I'll be using it for.
4. Add 1–2 Tbsp apple cider vinegar. This is optional but recommended because the vinegar helps extract the minerals from the bones, but it also makes the broth slightly less palatable so don't go overboard.
5. Add filtered water to the slow cooker until the bones are covered, leaving about an inch of room at the top.
6. Let it cook for at least 24 hours, ideally 48 or even longer!
7. Once you're ready to harvest your broth, pour it through a strainer into a pot or bowl and allow it to cool.
8. Use it or freeze it for later! (See How to Store Bone Broth).
9. When it cools it may have a thick layer of fat at the top. You can certainly eat it but sometimes I find it tough to digest so I skim it off and cook with it instead.
10. If you've used a good amount of bones, your broth will likely gel in the fridge. This is great! Don't fret if your broth doesn't gel after cooling. See Troubleshooting: Why didn't my broth gel? for more info.

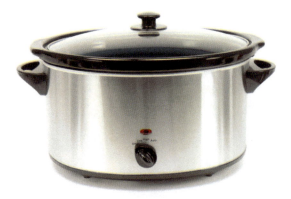

If you want to put the bones in for another round, by all means do it again. Sometimes we get 3 or 4 rounds worth of broth from one set of bones! You can cook the bones until they completely disintegrate and this way you are really getting your money's worth!

A twist on the slow cooker method is what my friend Jenny from NourishedKitchen.com calls Perpetual Bone Broth. I love this idea because it makes cooking bone broth even easier and lower maintenance and I'm all about saving time in the kitchen and saving dishes to wash.

Jenny recommends taking out 2 cups to a quart of broth from your slow cooker each day (after it's been cooking for 48 hours) and replacing it with filtered water. Keep doing this throughout the week and you'll always have bone broth on hand to add to your meals or sip in a mug!

A few notes on perpetual broth: If you don't take out 2 cups of broth each day it may take on a burnt flavor. Also, adding vegetables to your broth would not be recommended as the flavor can become too intense when cooked for so long. Make sure to keep your slow cooker filled with water to about an inch of the top.

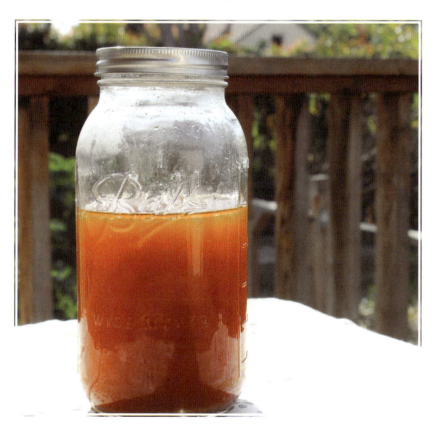

Pressure Cooker Method (fastest method, hands on)

This is a great method if you want to just get your broth making over with in one fell swoop during your weekend batch cooking day or on a day where you'll be home for several hours.

You can add vegetables to this one if you'd like since you won't be cooking it forever like in the previous method. Any vegetable will do but onions, carrots and celery are the most popular ones. I would hold off on the salt until you're ready to use the broth since it's easy for it to get out of hand since this will make a concentrated broth.

What you will need:

- Quality bones: as little or as many as you want — 2lbs is a good starting point, either frozen or thawed
- Filtered water
- 1–2 Tbsp Organic unfiltered Apple Cider Vinegar
- Pressure cooker

Pressure Cooker Directions:

1. Place your bones (about 2 lbs), vegetables and 1–2 Tbsp of apple cider vinegar into the pressure cooker.
2. Cover with filtered water until the ⅔ recommended fill point (varies depending on pressure cooker).
3. Close the valve and turn on high and place on a burner on high heat.
4. As soon as the pressure cooker indicates high pressure, turn it to low and cook for 30–40 minutes (not longer).
5. Remove from heat and let the pressure release on its own (about 10 minutes).
6. Strain in a mesh strainer over a bowl or pot.
7. Enjoy, use or store for later!

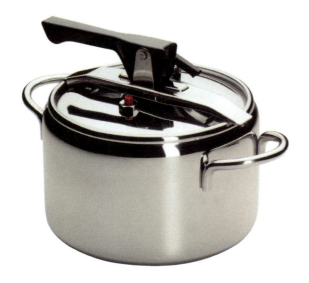

Regular Stock Pot Method (for the gadget averse)

If you don't have a slow cooker or pressure cooker, you'll be glad to know you can make bone broth the way your grandmother or great grandmother would have done it: in a regular stainless steel stock pot. I would recommend using the largest pot you have so you can make a big batch and freeze for later.

Depending on which bones you choose you'll have to simmer for different lengths of time.

* Beef, pork or lamb: 48 hours
* Chicken or Turkey: 24 hours
* Fish: 8 hours

What you will need:

* Quality bones: as little or as many as you want—2lbs is a good starting point, either frozen or thawed
* Filtered water
* 1–2 Tbsp Organic unfiltered Apple Cider Vinegar
* Stainless steel stock pot

Directions:

1. Place your bones (at least 2 lbs) in the stock pot with 1–2 Tbsp of apple cider vinegar
2. Cover with filtered water leaving an inch of room at the top.
3. Place the pot on high heat until it boils.
4. As soon as it boils, turn it to low heat and allow it to simmer for the recommended time depending on type of bones as mentioned above. You can skim the foam/impurities at the top as it's simmering if you'd like.
5. Allow it to cool and store. When it cools you may notice a layer of fat at the top. I'd recommend removing it. You can cook with it if you'd like, or discard it.
6. Enjoy, use it in a recipe, or store for later.

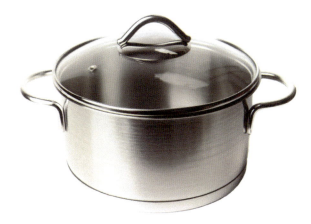

HOW TO STORE BONE BROTH

When putting mason jars in the freezer, always make sure that you leave room on the top! Otherwise, the jar might explode as the frozen broth expands.

Bone broth will keep in the fridge for about 1 week. You will know that it is near the end of its life when the gel starts to melt. In the freezer it will last about 6 months. Mason jars are probably the most popular way of storing bone broth.

Another option is to freeze the broth in ice cube trays. Then you can dump the broth cubes into a freezer bag and you'll always have small portions on hand. You can even cook these on the stove to reduce them further and get super-concentrated portions of broth which is especially useful for recipes like the Demi-Glace.

Storing bone broth in metal containers is *not* recommended. The gelatin might react with the metal and cause corrosion.

TROUBLESHOOTING: WHY DIDN'T MY BROTH GEL?

Bone broth is usually going to be gelatinous because of all of the collagen in it. If it doesn't gel, it is okay — the broth will still be full of nutrients from the bones, like magnesium, calcium, and phosphorus. But, if you want to get all of the amazing benefits of gelatin, you'll probably want your broth to gel. That's a sign it is super rich in gelatin.

There are 5 main reasons why your bone broth might not have gelled.[116]

1. You didn't use enough bones

If you don't use enough bones, then there might not be enough collagen to turn the water into a gel. Ideally, you should have a ratio of 1 pound of chicken bones to quart of water. Or, for beef or other ruminants, a ratio of 7 pounds bone to 4 quarts of water. If you don't feel like dealing with measurements, go by the rule that you should just add enough water to cover the bones completely.

2. You didn't use bones high in collagen

To get a jelly broth, you will need to use bones and parts which are rich in collagen. Chicken feet, necks and heads are great to use. For ruminants, try adding some knuckle bone. If you can find it, oxtail is rich in collagen and you can add it to the mix to make a very jelly broth. I usually add chicken feet or heads to my broth even if the rest of the bones are beef.

3. You used bones from CAFOs
(Concentrated Animal Feeding Operations)

A lot of people don't have luck making their broth gel when using low quality CAFO bones. One can only assume that these animals weren't able to develop strong joints because they were cooped up in tiny cages for their entire lives. Just one more reason why it is best to buy pastured animal bones! If you truly have absolutely no way to get your hands on or afford these high quality bones, you will still see some benefit from making broth than forgoing it all together. Just do the best you can, and upgrade to better quality bones when you are able to.

4. You let the temperature get too high

Once your bone broth has come to a boil, you will need to promptly turn down the heat to its lowest setting so it simmers, not boils. If you let it boil at high temperatures, then the heat will destroy the collagen!

5. You didn't let the broth cook for long enough

As mentioned earlier, beef/ruminant bones should ideally be simmered for 48 hours, chicken for 24 hours, and fish for 8 hours. If you simmer the bones for less than this, the collagen won't have time to be drawn from the bones. If you don't add apple cider vinegar to the bones/water (which helps draw the collagen out), then you will definitely need to cook the bones longer before it gels.

If your broth doesn't gel and you just want to get some more gelatin into your diet, you can always dissolve a couple tablespoons of quality gelatin powder into it (see the resource page) and that will certainly make it gel.

So, now you've got all this gelatin-rich bone broth? What are you supposed to do with it?

I have come to love sipping a mug of bone broth, especially in the cold months. But I understand that not everyone loves the taste of bone broth as much as I do! In the following savory recipes, you will find all sorts of recipes for how you can use bone broth in your daily life. The more the merrier!

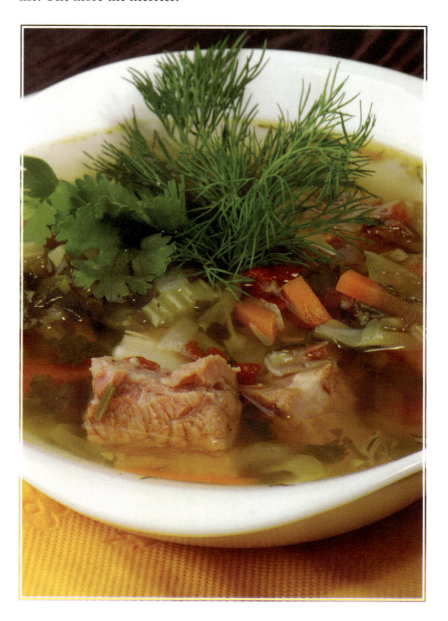

Side Dish Recipes

In the following pages you'll find some ideas for side dishes where you can generously use bone broth. These are just a few ideas to get you started.

You can pretty much use bone broth wherever you would normally use water, as in the recipe for Sauteéd Chard, where, even though the liquid will evaporate the minerals will remain behind adding nutrients and flavor to your dish. You can also use it in purées such as the Pumpkin Purée and the Root Veggie Mash.

Even in recipes where your need for liquid is minimal, just adding a bit of bone broth is helpful! Experiment to see just how many meals you can get it into.

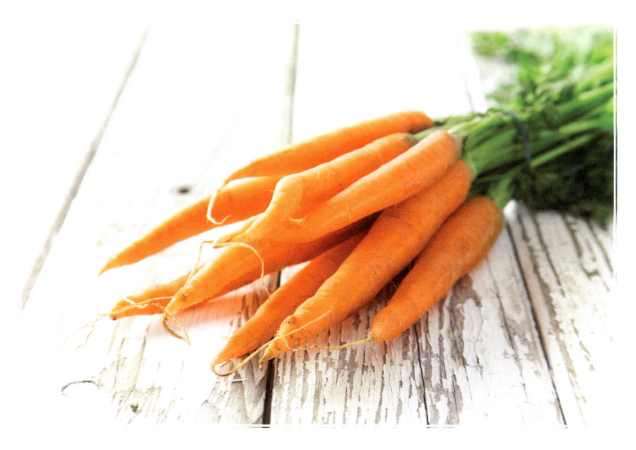

PUMPKIN PURÉE

What you will need:

- 2 cups cooked pumpkin (you can use canned pumpkin too!)
- 6 Tbsp. ghee
- ¼ cup bone broth
- ½ tsp. sea salt
- dash of pepper, cinnamon

Directions:

1. If using fresh pumpkin, cut it in half and lay it (skin up) on a large baking dish or roasting pan. Add about 1 inch of water. Bake at 375 for 1 hour or until flesh is soft. Remove 2 cups flesh for the recipe. The rest you can freeze for later or use in another recipe.
2. Mix all ingredients together in a pot
3. Let the mash simmer while stirring until you get the desired consistency
4. Enjoy!

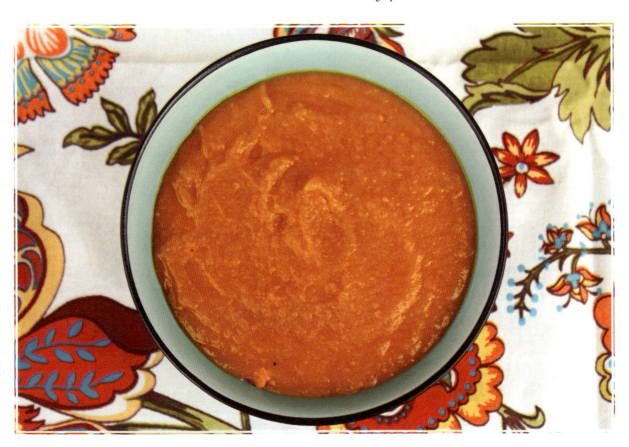

BRAISED BRUSSELS SPROUTS WITH BACON

Ingredients:

- 6 cups Brussels sprouts (halved)
- 1 ½ cups bone broth
- 1 Tbsp. coconut oil
- salt and pepper to taste

Directions:

1. Place sprouts in a large baking dish with broth
2. Bake at 375 degrees for 1 hour
3. While baking cook 1 pound of bacon
4. When finished, crumble bacon and add to sprouts with coconut oil
5. Enjoy!

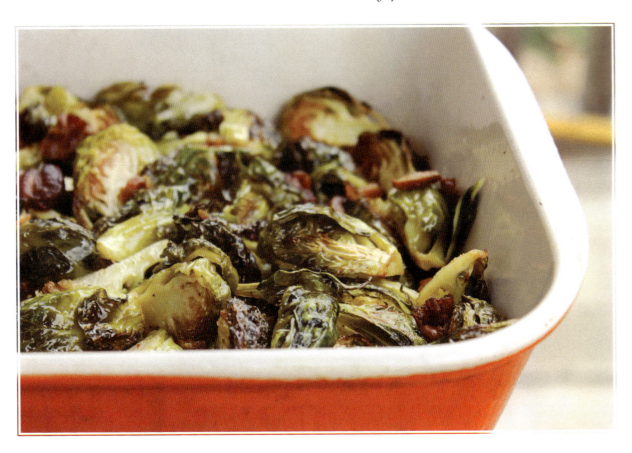

SAUTEÉD CHARD

Ingredients:

- 1 large bunch of chard
- ¼ cup bone broth
- 2 cloves garlic
- Juice from 1 lemon
- Sea salt and pepper to taste

Directions:

1. Place pre-chopped chard in large pot
2. Add bone broth
3. Bring to a simmer on medium heat
4. Let simmer for 7 minutes
5. Add garlic (crushed) and lemon
6. Let simmer for 3 more minutes
7. Sea salt and pepper to taste
8. Enjoy!

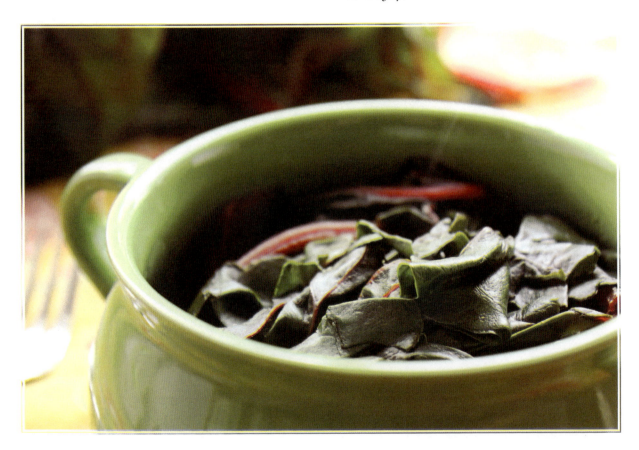

GLAZED CARROTS

Ingredients:

- 2 bags/bunches organic carrots
- 2 cups bone broth
- 1 tsp. cinnamon
- 2 tsp. sea salt

Directions:

1. Wash your carrots and cut into 1 inch long sections
2. Place in a roasting pan with bone broth
3. Add salt and cinnamon
4. Cover with lid and bake for 1 hour and 15 minutes at 350 degrees
5. Enjoy!

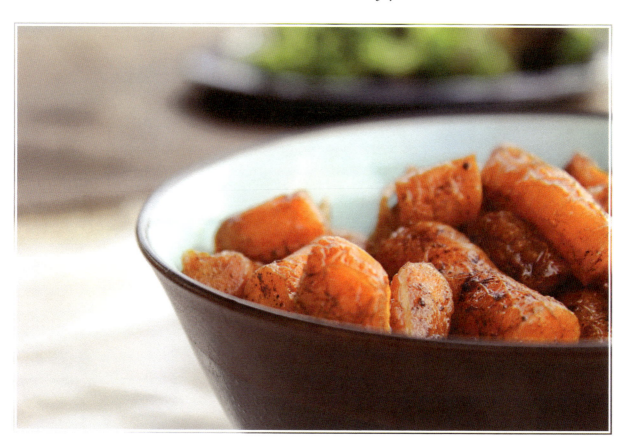

ROOT VEGGIE MASH

Ingredients:

- 2 cups bone broth
- 5 carrots
- 4 small sweet potatoes
- 3 turnips
- 1 beet
- Cream from 1 can of coconut milk
- ¼ cup ghee
- 2 tsp. sea salt
- 1 tsp. pepper

Directions:

1. Bake your washed and skinned veggies in a roasting pan with 1 cup of the bone broth at 350 degrees for 1 hour
2. Remove veggies from oven and place them into a pot with the remaining bone broth and other ingredients
3. Heat on low
4. Use an immersion blender to blend the mixture
5. Enjoy!

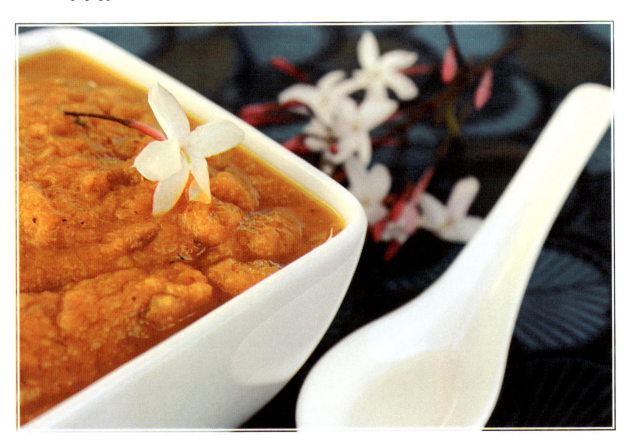

Soups

Soups are perhaps the most obvious use for bone broth. I like to make a big batch of soup to have in the fridge for the whole week. Even just a small serving of soup as a complement to your dinner every night is a great, no-hassle way to get a hefty amount of bone broth into your diet. After a couple of weeks it will become addictive and you'll feel as if it's not a proper meal without your cup of soup!

In many cultures, soup is a breakfast staple. It may seem odd to us westerners but really it's just a matter of what we're used to. When I started having soup for breakfast I realized it was probably the easiest, most nutrient dense food I could start my day with. It also solved the problem of "I no longer eat cereal for breakfast; what on earth can I eat that's easy to simply pour in a bowl in the morning?!". Easy peasy.

Here are 5 soup recipes to get you started. No need to buy expensive, junk-ridden canned soups. Make a big batch on the weekend, freeze some of it and eat the rest throughout the week! Your body will thank you for it.

CHICKEN SOUP

Ingredients:

- 5 cups chicken bone broth
- 5 cups filtered water
- 1 lb chopped chicken meat
- 1 bunch carrots
- 2 medium onions
- 1 bunch celery
- 2 tbsp. sea salt

Optional: if you've just gotta have some noodles in your chicken soup but you're grain-free, use a spiral slicer to whip up some zucchini noodles to toss in! Delicious and easy!

Directions:

1. Combine the bone broth and water in a large pot.
2. Heat on medium until simmering.
3. Chop onions, carrots and celery and add to pot.
4. Add chicken.
5. Heat until simmering again.
6. Add salt.
7. Let simmer until veggies are soft.
8. Enjoy!

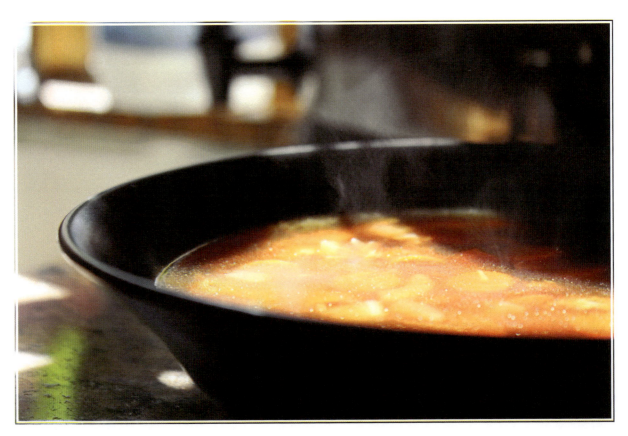

CREAMY BUTTERNUT SQUASH SOUP

Ingredients:

- 2 cups bone broth
- 1 large butternut squash
- 13.5oz (1 can) full-fat coconut milk
- 1 large onion
- ½ bunch of Swiss chard
- ¼ cup ghee or butter (preferably grass-fed)
- 2 tsp. sea salt
- ½ tsp. pepper

Directions:

1. Cut the squash in half and place (skin up) in a pan filled with 1 inch of water. Put the squash in the oven at 375 degrees for 1 hour and 15 minutes
2. Steam the chard
3. Sauté the onions until translucent and set aside
4. Once the squash is ready, remove the seeds and put what remains into a large pot on low heat
5. Add the remaining ingredients and blend with an immersion blender
6. Let cook until the desired consistency
7. Add salt and pepper as needed
8. Enjoy!

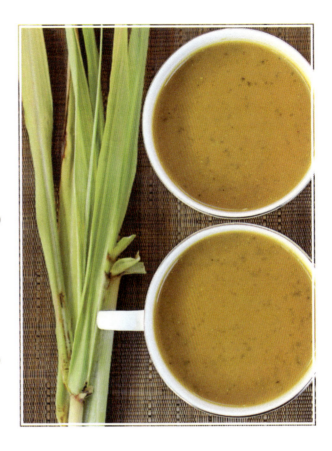

SWEET POTATO SOUP

Ingredients:

- 4 cups bone broth (I used chicken)
- 13.5oz (1 can) full-fat coconut milk
- 1 cup filtered water
- 2 large sweet potatoes
- 1 large onion
- ¼ cup ghee or butter (preferably grass-fed)
- 2 ½ tsp. sea salt
- ½ tsp. pepper

Directions:

1. Put the sweet potatoes in the oven at 375 degrees for 1 hour (poke them with a fork first so they don't explode!)
2. Sauté the onion and set aside
3. Once the sweet potatoes are easy to pierce with a fork or knife, peel them and put them in a pot
4. Add the onions and remaining ingredients
5. Mix well with an immersion blender
6. Bring to a boil and let simmer for 20 minutes
7. Enjoy!

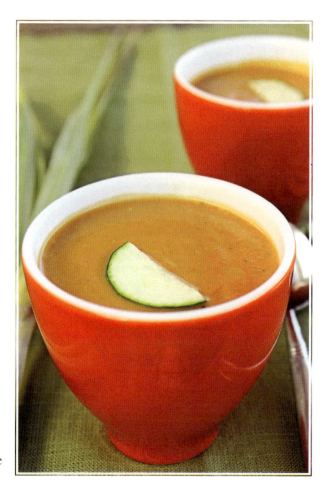

CREAM OF CHICKEN SOUP WITH LEMONGRASS

Ingredients:

- 6 cups chicken bone broth
- 27oz (2 cans) full-fat coconut milk
- 1 cup shredded chicken
- 6 shoots of lemongrass
- 1 ½ tsp sea salt
- ½ tsp. pepper

Directions:

1. Bring the bone broth with shredded chicken to a boil
2. Add coconut milk, salt, and pepper
3. Mix with an immersion blender
4. Once blended add the lemongrass
5. Let simmer for 45 minutes
6. Enjoy!

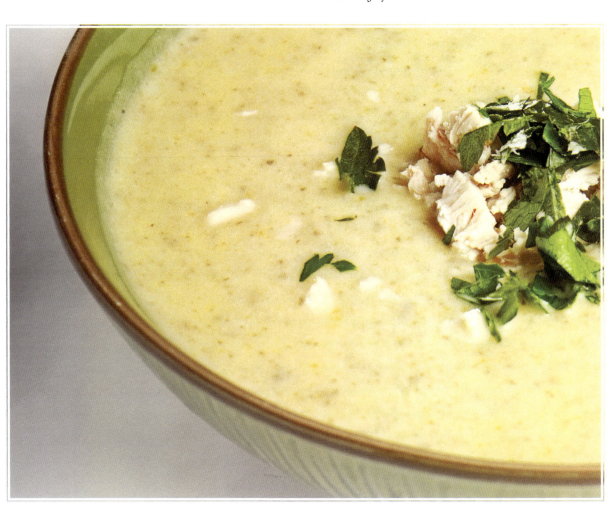

"TORTILLA" SOUP

Ingredients:

- 4 cups bone broth (I used chicken)
- 13.5oz (1 can) full-fat coconut milk
- 2 tomatoes (chopped) or 1 can stewed tomatoes (strained)
- 1 yellow onion (minced)
- 1 red bell pepper (chopped)
- Juice from 2 medium sized limes
- 3 cloves of garlic (minced)
- 2 Tbsp coconut oil
- 1 tsp cumin
- 1 Tbsp sea salt
- 1 tsp pepper
- Dash of red pepper

Garnish:

- Plantain chips
- Sliced avocado
- Fresh cilantro

Directions:

1. Pour bone broth in a large pot and turn heat to medium
2. Add ingredients to pot and bring to a boil
3. Stir occasionally
4. Let simmer for 30 minutes
5. Reduce heat
6. Use immersion blender to blend the soup
7. If the soup is too watery, continue to simmer until you get the consistency you want
8. Add salt as needed
9. Garnish with plantain chips, avocado and a fresh sprig of cilantro
10. Enjoy!

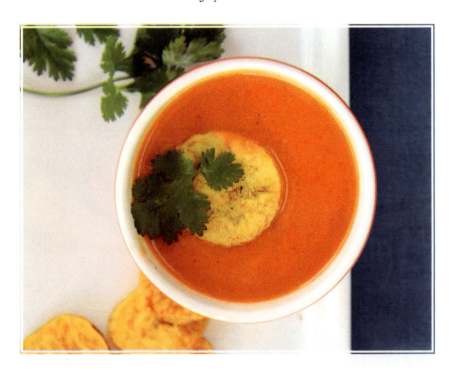

Condiments and Sauces

If you've got picky eaters at home or if bone broth is totally new to you, this is a great way to sneak it into your diet! Adding bone broth to your homemade sauces and condiments makes them not only delicious but nutrient dense as well.

Store-bought condiments, even the organic ones, are often laden with preservatives and sugars. Of course, it's much better to buy an organic ketchup that has organic sugar in it than the conventional one full of genetically modified organisms (GMOs) and high fructose corn syrup. I still buy them in a pinch since I don't always get around to making condiments myself, but I use them as an occasional treat more than a staple.

By contrast, the recipes included here I use liberally when we have them on hand and I encourage my kids to help themselves as they are not only free of junk, they are also chock full of healthy fats and nutrient dense broth. Go ahead and serve yourself a big helping. You have my blessing.

KETCHUP

Ingredients:

- 1 cup tomato paste
- 1 cup bone broth
- ½ cup maple syrup
- 2 tsp salt
- 1 tsp garlic powder
- ½ tsp. paprika
- ½ tsp pepper

Directions:

1. Combine all ingredients into a small pot on med/low heat
2. Use an immersion blender to blend ingredients until smooth
3. Add bone broth if needed to get desired consistency
4. Let cool and place in fridge
5. Re-fill your expensive organic ketchup bottle and your kids won't know the difference!

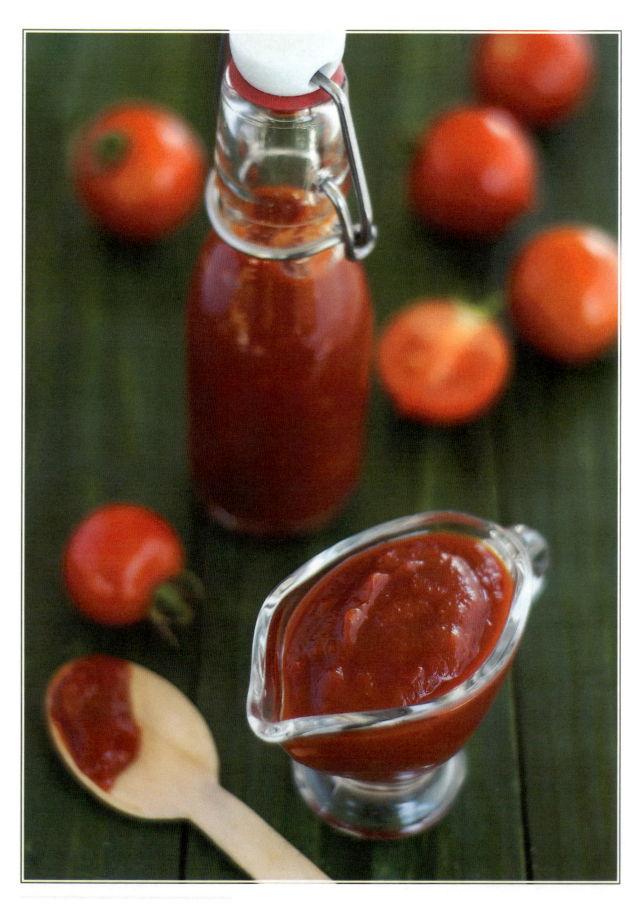

MAYONNAISE

What you will need:

- Food processor or a whisk and some stamina
- 1 cup coconut oil
- 2 large egg yolks
- 1 Tbsp. lemon juice
- 2 tsp. apple cider vinegar
- 1 tsp. gluten free mustard
- ½ tsp salt (add more later to taste if needed)
- 1 Tbsp. Gelatin (green packaging)

Directions:

1. Combine the egg yolk, lemon juice, vinegar, mustard and salt in a food processor or bowl.
2. Mix until blended and bright yellow.
3. Use the drip function on the food processor to slowly add the coconut oil while the processor is mixing or add ¼ tsp. at a time while whisking by hand.
4. Mix until you get the consistency you want — it will not be as solidified as store-bought mayo, but it will be spreadable once it spends some time in the fridge.
5. Enjoy!

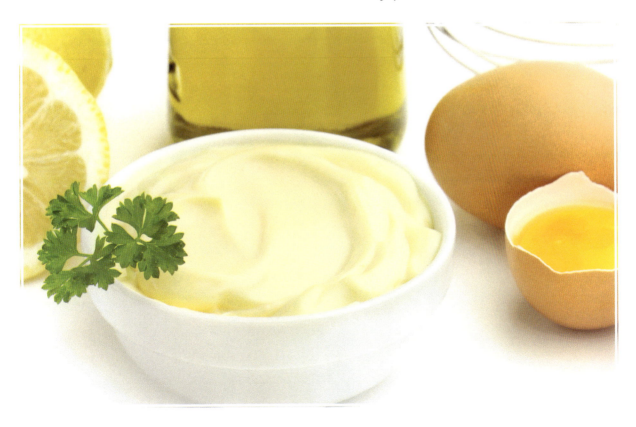

BBQ SAUCE

Ingredients:

- 1 cup bone broth (I used chicken)
- ¼ cup coconut nectar
- ¼ cup pomegranate molasses
- ¼ cup coconut aminos
- ⅛ cup apple cider vinegar
- 1 small can organic tomato paste
- 1 tsp. garlic powder

Directions:

1. Combine all ingredients in sauce pan over med/low heat
2. Use an immersion blender to mix sauce
3. Turn off heat and let cool
4. Enjoy!

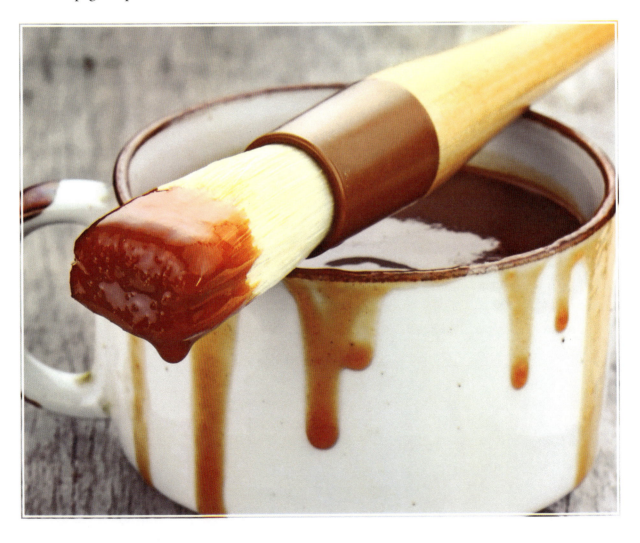

DEMI-GLACE

Ingredients:

- 4 cups bone broth

Directions:

1. Filter bone broth through a fine mesh filter
2. Pour into a medium size pot
3. Turn heat to medium and bring to a simmer
4. Mix periodically
5. Let reduce until you have around 1 cup
6. Turn off heat
7. Enjoy!

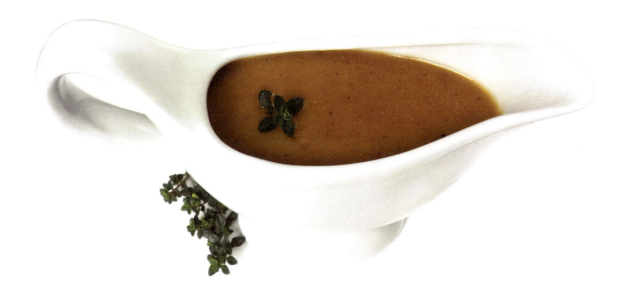

GRAVY

Ingredients:

- ½ cup beef/pork/chicken fat left over from cooled bone broth (scrape from top)
- 3 cups chicken or turkey bone broth
- 1 yellow onion (diced)
- 1 Tbsp. ghee or coconut oil
- 1 tsp. dried sage
- ½ tsp. pepper
- Sea salt to taste

Directions:

1. Put fat in sauce-pan and add chopped onion
2. Cook for 15 minutes on med/high or until onion is translucent
3. Add remaining ingredients and bring to a boil
4. Reduce heat to simmer
5. Use an immersion blender to mix ingredients
6. Let simmer until gravy reduces to an appropriate consistency
7. Salt to taste
8. Enjoy!

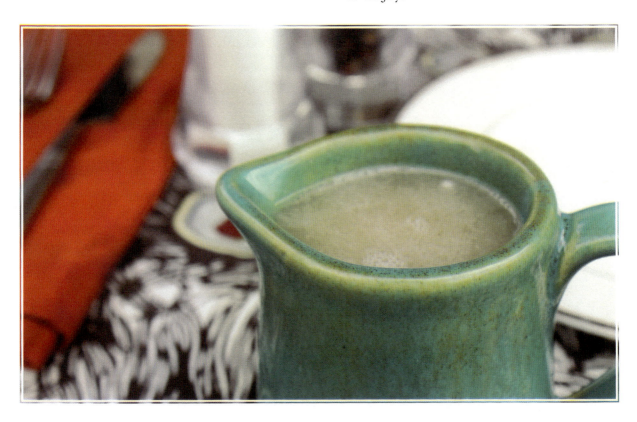

"Jello" Recipes

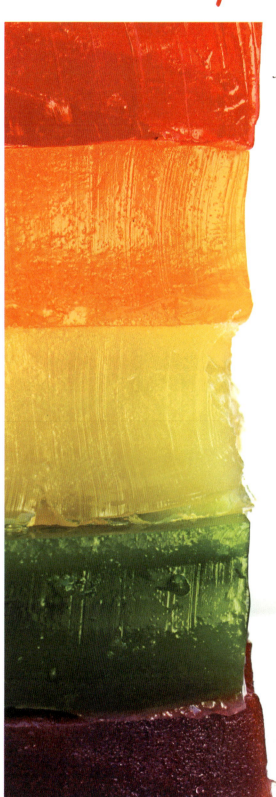

Finally, the recipes which gelatin is best known for! Jell-O has been a staple hospital food for many years. It has been a popular kid snack for just as long and most of us probably remember the Bill Cosby commercial campaign featuring this popular food.

Of course, we now know that Jell-O was just junk food that not only didn't nourish our bodies, it served up a nice dose of food coloring, sugar, and other additives.

Let's give Jell-O a makeover. Here are several recipes to do just that. If you like to have a treat after dinner each night but don't have time to make one from scratch, these are great recipes to make on a weekend and have on hand to serve throughout the week.

Make sure you use the *red* packaging of Great Lakes gelatin and NOT the green one which says collagen hydrolysate. Only the one labeled gelatin will gel!

ORANGE JELLO

Ingredients:

- 2 cups orange juice (ideally fresh squeezed and strained)
- 2 Tbsp. gelatin

Directions:

1. Pour ½ cup of orange juice into saucepan on low heat.
2. Pour in your gelatin and mix well until dissolved.
3. Pour in the remaining juice and turn off heat.
4. Pour into gelatin into a glass bowl or several small bowls.
5. Let cool and place in the fridge for at least 3 hours.
6. Enjoy!

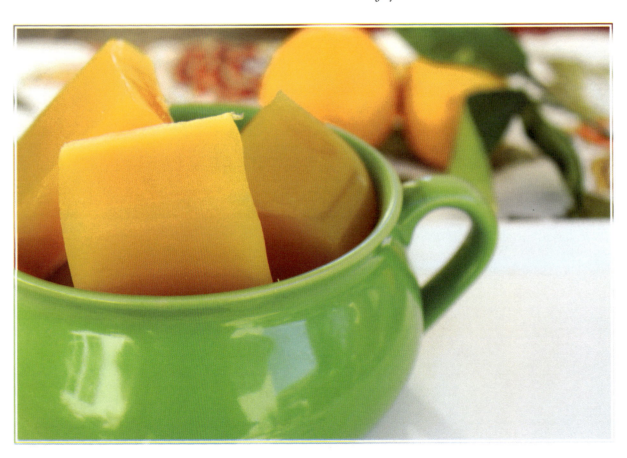

STRAWBERRY JELLO

Ingredients:

- 2 ½ cups pureed strawberries (roughly 4 small baskets if using fresh)
- 1 cup filtered water
- ½ cup maple syrup (preferably organic grade B)
- ¼ cup lemon juice
- 3 Tbsp gelatin

Directions:

1. Purée the strawberries in the food processor or blender until fully blended
2. Pour all ingredients (excluding gelatin) into a pot
3. Heat on medium until warm, then turn down to low
4. Use an immersion blender to mix ingredients
5. Add gelatin and mix well with the immersion blender
6. Pour into a pan or jello mold
7. Let cool
8. Place in fridge for 2 hours
9. Enjoy!

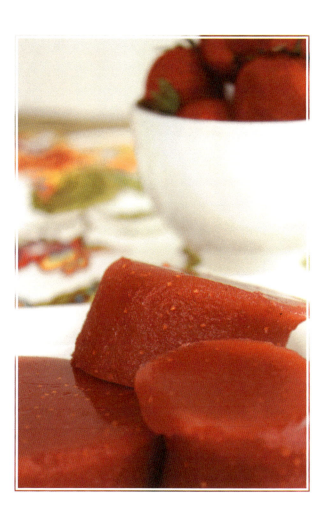

BLUEBERRY JELLO

Ingredients:

- 3 cups blueberries
- 2 cups filtered water
- ½ cup maple syrup (preferably organic grade B)
- ⅛ cup lemon juice
- 3 Tbsp gelatin

Directions:

1. Pour water and blueberries into a large pot and bring to a boil
2. Use an immersion blender to mash the blueberries and water
3. Strain the mixture and put back in the pot
4. Add syrup and lemon juice
5. Add 3 Tbsp gelatin and mix well with the immersion blender
6. Pour into a pan or jello mold
7. Let cool
8. Place in fridge for 2 hours
9. Enjoy!

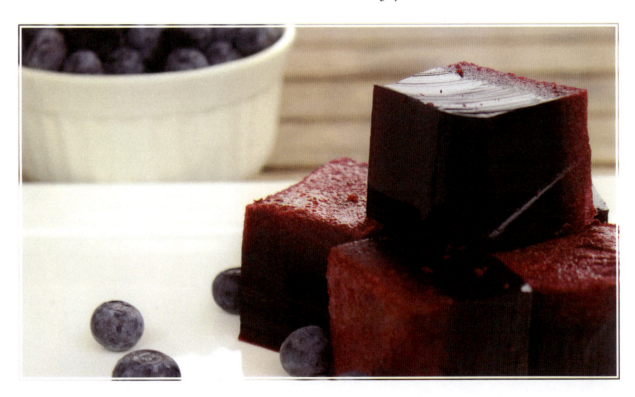

LEMON JELLO

Ingredients:

- 1 cup lemon juice
- ½ cup maple syrup (preferably organic grade B)
- ¾ cup filtered water
- 3 Tbsp gelatin

Directions:

1. Pour all ingredients (excluding gelatin) into a pot
2. Heat on medium until warm, then turn down to low
3. Use an immersion blender to mix ingredients
4. Add gelatin and mix well with the immersion blender
5. Pour into a pan or jello mold
6. Let cool
7. Place in fridge for 2 hours
8. Enjoy!

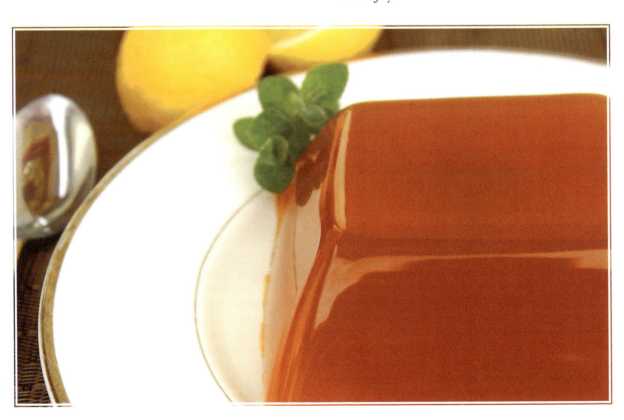

HIBISCUS TEA JELLO

Ingredients:

- 3 cups hibiscus tea
- ⅛ cup lemon juice
- ¼ cup maple syrup (preferably organic grade B)
- 3 Tbsp. Gelatin

Directions:

1. Brew hibiscus tea
2. Pour all ingredients (excluding gelatin) into a pot
3. Heat on medium until warm, then turn down to low
4. Use an immersion blender to mix ingredients
5. Add gelatin and mix well with the immersion blender
6. Pour into a pan or jello mold
7. Let cool
8. Place in fridge for 2 hours
9. Enjoy!

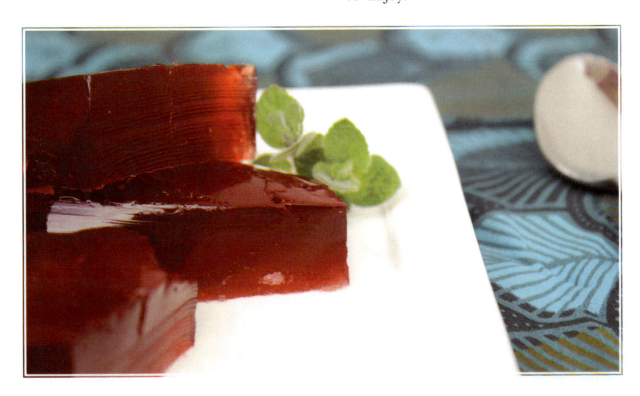

KOMBUCHA JELLO

For those who don't know, kombucha is a probiotic drink made from sweet tea. This tea is left to ferment and, because it contains all sorts of good bacteria, it is great for balancing your gut flora. As we talked about earlier in the gut health section, gut health is linked to everything from weight to mood. You can easily make your own kombucha (read my instructions on my website here) or you can buy kombucha too. On the resource page, you can find recommendations for my favorite brands of gut-healthy kombucha.

Ingredients:

- 2 cups kombucha in the flavor of your choice
- 2 Tbsp gelatin
- 1 Tbsp maple syrup (preferably organic grade B) (optional)

Directions:

1. Pour kombucha and maple syrup into a pot
2. Heat on low until warm
3. Mix ingredients
4. Add gelatin and mix well with the immersion blender
5. Pour into a pan or jello mold
6. Let cool
7. Place in fridge for 2 hours
8. Enjoy!

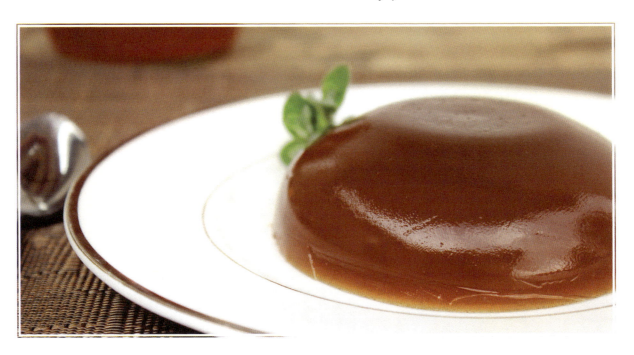

Gummies

Gummies pack a hefty dose of gelatin, are easy to make in large batches and keep really well for weeks at a time. Of course, in my house they last about 10 minutes so if you plan on keeping them around, I recommend hiding them from kids and adults alike.

I love having gummies on hand to pack in my kids' lunches, hand out as an after dinner treat and take to work with me to have on hand when I want a treat. The fact that they're delicious and super nutrient dense as well is a win-win.

These recipes use mostly whole fruit. This is a small additional step, requiring pureeing or juicing, but I find it really makes a difference in the taste and quality of ingredients used. If you'd like to cut a corner and buy a fruit juice instead, you can certainly do that, just read labels carefully and try to find the cleanest one you can (with the least amount of ingredients, all of which you can pronounce). Finding an additive free juice is probably impossible unless you're buying fresh squeezed but you can probably easily find an organic, unsweetened version to use. Of course, they will likely be pricier.

Just do the best you can. As I mentioned in the broth section, when it comes to ingredients quality is important but it's also about making the best choices you can within your budget and based on availability. Improve when and where you can later.

STRAWBERRY LEMONADE GUMMIES

What you will need:

- 1 cup pureed strawberries
- ⅓ cup lemon juice
- 7 Tbsp. gelatin
- 2 Tbsp. honey (preferably raw)
- Silicone molds

Directions:

1. Pour strawberry mixture, lemon juice and honey into a pan on low/medium heat.
2. Mix well until warm (not hot as it will kill the awesome probiotic properties of the raw honey!).
3. Add gelatin and mix well until dissolved.
4. Pour contents of pan into a cup with a spout (like a measuring cup).
5. Pour mixture into candy molds.
6. Place in freezer for 15 minutes. For easy transport, place the silicone mold on a cookie sheet.
7. Enjoy!

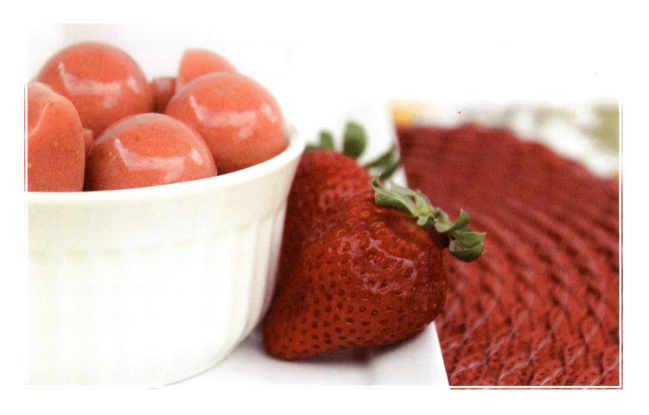

STRAWBERRY CREAM GUMMIES

What you will need:

- Immersion blender
- 13.5oz (1 can) full-fat coconut milk
- 1 cup of pureed strawberries
- ¼ cup maple syrup (preferably organic grade B)
- ¼ cup lemon juice
- 13 Tbsp gelatin
- 4 Tbsp honey (preferably raw)
- 2 Tbsp vanilla
- Silicone molds

Directions:

1. Combine strawberries, lemon juice and honey on low heat in a small pot on the stove.
2. Stir until warm, not hot as it will kill the probiotic quality in the honey.
3. Add 7 Tbsp gelatin and immediately mix with an immersion blender until smooth and lump free.
4. Pour strawberry mixture into your molds, but ONLY fill each one half way (the rest of the space will be filled by the cream).
5. Put the strawberry molds into the freezer. For easy transport, place the silicone mold on a cookie sheet.
6. Combine the coconut milk, vanilla and maple syrup and warm on low.
7. Add 6 Tbsp gelatin and mix immediately with immersion blender.
8. Take out strawberry molds and complete the pouring with the cream portion.
9. Put back in the freezer for 30 minutes
10. Bring out and let sit until room temperature
11. Enjoy!

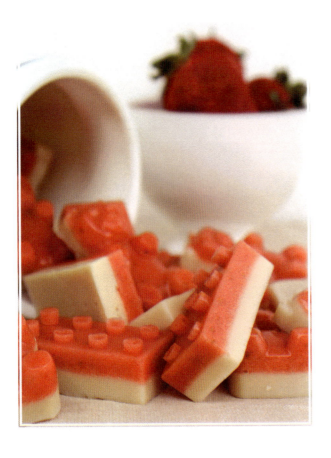

LEMON GUMMIES

What you will need:

* ⅓ cup fresh squeezed lemon juice
* 3 Tbsp gelatin
* 2 Tbsp honey (preferably raw)
* Silicone molds

Directions:

1. Pour lemon juice and honey into a skillet on low heat
2. Once warm (not hot since it will kill the probiotic awesomeness of the raw honey!) mix in the gelatin.
3. Mix thoroughly until the gelatin has dissolved.
4. Pour into a measuring cup, and then into molds
5. Put in freezer for 15 minutes (for easy transport, place the silicone mold on a cookie sheet).
6. Take out and enjoy!

* *If you or your kids are used to sweeter foods you may want to start with more and as time goes by you can experiment with reducing the quantity*

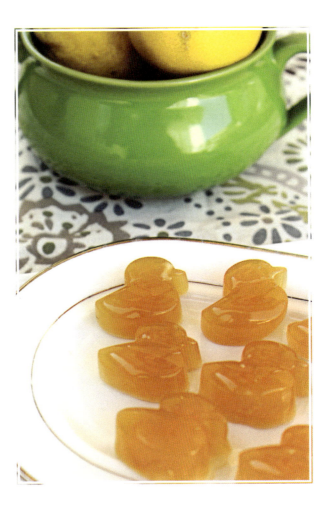

ORANGE GUMMY BEARS

What you will need:

- ⅓ cup of fresh-squeezed orange juice
- 3 Tbsp Gelatin
- 2–3 Tbsp honey (preferably raw)
- Silicone molds

Directions:

1. Combine all the ingredients on a pot on low heat
2. Heat it up enough to dissolve it, stirring constantly (but don't boil it because you'll kill the awesome probiotic qualities in the raw honey).
3. Pour into silicone molds.
4. Place in the freezer for 10 minutes (for easy transport, place the silicone mold on a cookie sheet).
5. Take out and enjoy!

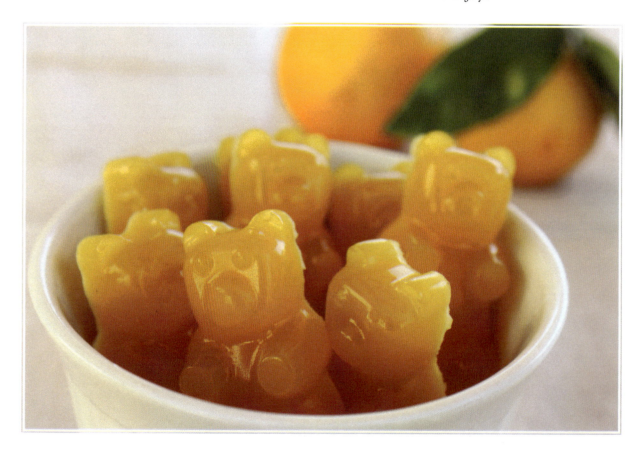

BLUEBERRY GUMMIES

What you will need:

- 1 cup pureed blueberries
- ¼ cup lemon juice
- 6 Tbsp. gelatin
- 4 Tbsp. honey (preferably raw)
- Silicone molds

Directions:

1. Mix all ingredients (excluding gelatin) in a pot and let simmer on low heat
2. Once mixed well, add gelatin and mix quickly with an immersion blender
3. Pour into molds and put in freezer for 20 minutes (for easy transport, place the silicone mold on a cookie sheet).
4. Take out and enjoy!

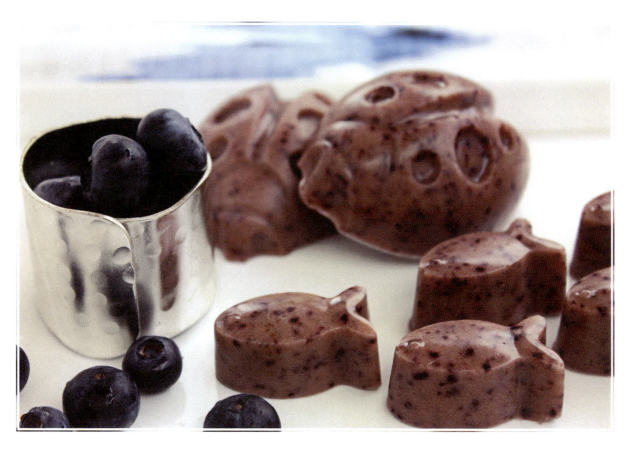

TANGERINE GUMMIES

What you will need:

- 1 cup strained (no pulp) tangerine juice
- 7 Tbsp gelatin
- 4 Tbsp honey (preferably raw)
- Silicone molds

Directions:

1. Bring the juice and honey to a low simmer (don't let it get too hot as it will kill the probiotic awesomeness of the honey!).
2. Add the gelatin and mix quickly with an immersion blender.
3. Pour into molds and place in freezer for 20 minutes (for easy transport, place the silicone mold on a cookie sheet).
4. Take out and enjoy!

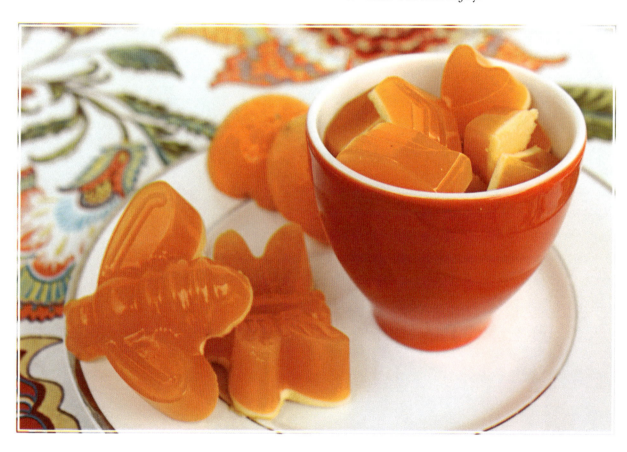

Dairy Free Ice Creams

Gelatin in Ice Cream? Adding gelatin to ice cream not only helps prevent the ice cream from freezing hard as a rock, but also has the bonus getting more nutrients into your diet! Have you noticed that store bought ice cream, even the cleanest brands, have junky emulsifiers like soy lecithin, guar gum, xanthan gum, carageenan and other strange ingredients? These ingredients help the ice cream have a creamier, easier to scoop consistency. Collagen hydrolysate, the form of gelatin that is water soluble (the green can), can do just that! It gives the ice cream a fluffier consistency and once you put in the freezer and take it out later you won't need an ice pick to get into it.

Now, I'm not necessarily prescribing a daily pint of ice cream for gut healing or anything but wanted to show you that ice cream is just one more thing you can use gelatin for. In the following pages you will find a few recipes for you to try. They are all dairy-free but, if you are not dairy intolerant, you could of course use milk in these recipes instead of coconut milk. If you do, I would highly recommend you use raw (unpasteurized) grass-fed milk if it is available in your area.

Experiment with your own concoctions! It's tough to get it wrong when it's just going in the freezer so use any fruit, or even vegetable you'd like.

MANGO ICE CREAM

What you will need:

- 3 ripe mangos
- 27oz (2 cans) full-fat coconut milk
- ¼ cup maple syrup (preferably grade B organic)
- 2 egg yolks
- 4 Tbsp Collagen Hydrolysate (the green can of gelatin which doesn't gel)
- 1 Tbsp. Vanilla
- Food processor or blender
- Ice cream maker

Directions:

1. Slice all three mangos and combine with coconut milk in food processor.
2. Add syrup, egg yolks, vanilla and gelatin.
3. Mix until smooth.
4. Add to the ice cream maker for roughly 30 minutes.
5. Enjoy!

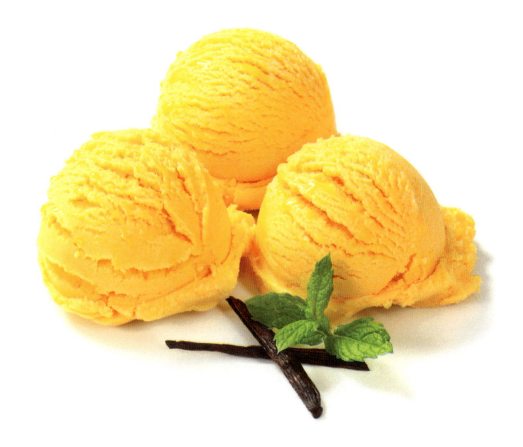

LEMON ICE CREAM

What you will need:

- 27oz (2 cans) full-fat coconut milk
- 3 egg yolks
- ¾ cup maple syrup (preferably grade B organic)
- ½ cup fresh lemon juice
- 4 Tbsp Collagen Hydrolysate (the green can of gelatin which doesn't gel)
- 1 ½ Tbsp grated lemon zest
- 1 tsp. vanilla
- Pinch of salt
- Ice cream maker

Directions:

1. In a pan mix together the zest, juice, maple syrup and eggs.
2. Add ½ can coconut milk, vanilla and gelatin.
3. Cook on medium heat stirring regularly until it comes to a simmer.
4. Turn off and let cool.
5. Once cool, strain the mixture, cover and place in the fridge until cold.
6. Once cold, add in the remainder of the coconut milk and mix well.
7. Place in your ice cream maker and let mix for 30–45 minutes.
8. Enjoy!

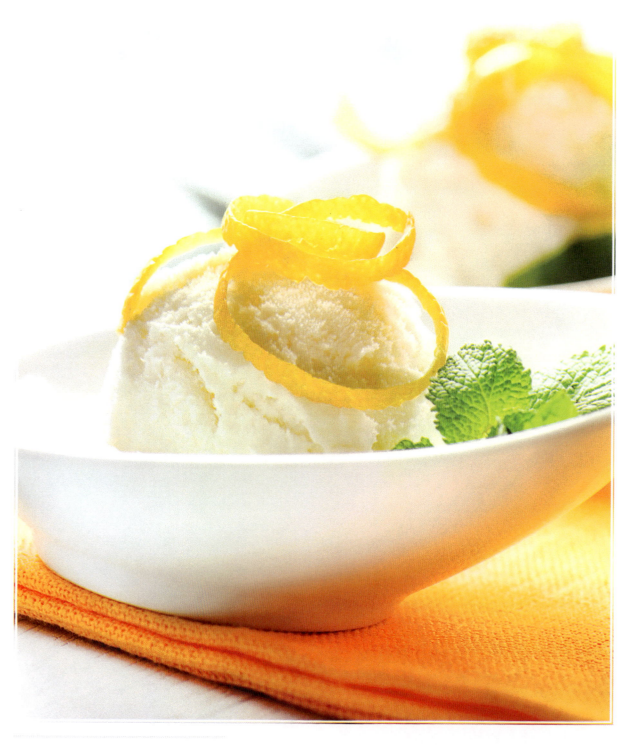

MAPLE BANANA ICE CREAM

Ingredients:

- 1 ½ cups banana
- 27oz (2 cans) full-fat coconut milk
- ½ cup maple syrup (preferably grade B organic)
- 2 egg yolks from pastured chickens
- 4 Tbsp Collagen Hydrolysate (the green can of gelatin which doesn't gel)
- 1 Tbsp vanilla extract
- Ice cream maker

Directions:

1. Blend all ingredients well in a food processor or blender.
2. Pour into the ice cream maker.
3. Let mix for about 30 minutes.
4. Put in freezer for harder ice cream, eat now for soft serve!

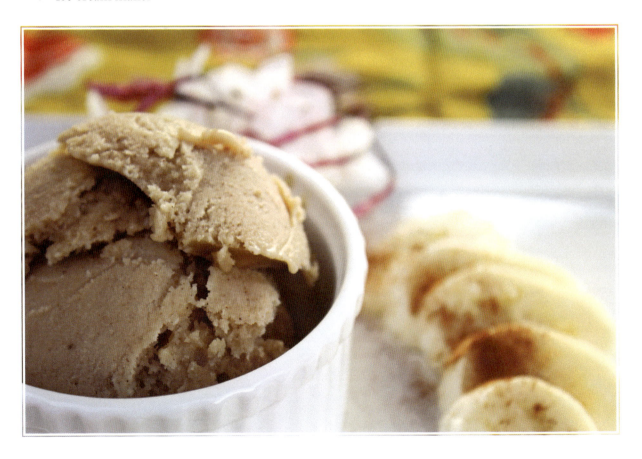

STRAWBERRY ICE CREAM

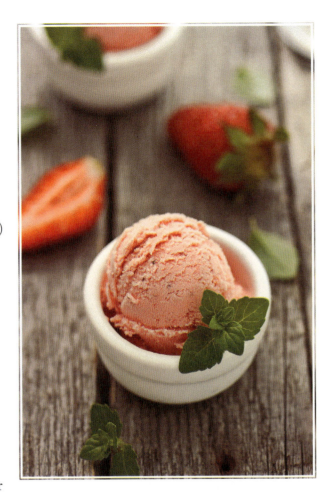

What you will need:

- 27oz (2 cans) full-fat coconut milk
- 3 egg yolks, preferably pastured
- 1 ½ cups strawberries (puréed)
- ½ cup maple syrup (preferably grade B organic)
- 4 Tbsp Collagen Hydrolysate (the green can of gelatin which doesn't gel)
- 1 Tbsp vanilla extract
- Ice cream maker

Directions:

1. Put all ingredients in a blender or food processor and mix well.
2. Pour into the ice cream maker.
3. Let mix 30 minutes.
4. Either transfer to a freezer safe container and put in the freezer for a few hours to harden more or eat right away for soft serve!
5. Enjoy!

VANILLA CHOCOLATE CHIP ICE CREAM

What you will need:

- 27oz (2 cans) full-fat coconut milk
- 2 egg yolks
- ½ cup maple syrup (preferably grade B organic)
- ¼ cup chocolate chips (I use Enjoy Life brand)
- 4 Tbsp Collagen Hydrolysate (the green can of gelatin which doesn't gel)
- 1 Tbsp vanilla
- Ice cream maker

Directions:

1. Mix the coconut milk, eggs, gelatin, vanilla and maple syrup in a blender or with an immersion blender for approximately 2 minutes or until blended well.
2. Pour the contents into your ice cream maker and turn on for 20 minutes.
3. Add the chocolate chips and let run for another 10 minutes.
4. Turn off and empty contents into an airtight container and place in the freezer for approximately 3 hours.
5. Take out and enjoy!

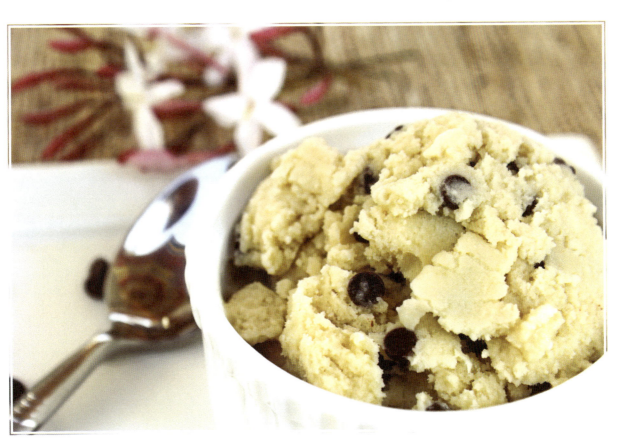

Dairy Free Smoothies

Another easy and quick way to start your morning, especially if the thought of having soup for breakfast sounds insane, is with a smoothie! Although gelatin is not a 100% complete protein, I would opt for using gelatin in your smoothie instead of protein powders, most of which are full of chemicals and highly processed sweeteners and additives.

Gelatin will not only keep you from feeling hungry, but it will also work to nourish your body in all the ways we discussed throughout the book.

A smoothie is also a great afternoon snack that grownups and kids alike will enjoy.

Here are a few ideas to get you started. Feel free to adapt your own favorite recipes or experiment with any fruits (and vegetables!) you like.

I've kept the recipes here dairy free. You could of course use raw (unpasteurized) grass-fed milk in place of coconut milk. If you want to use almond milk, look for one without emulsifiers or additives.

CHOCOLATE BANANA SMOOTHIE

Ingredients:

- ½ cup full-fat coconut milk
- ½ cup ice
- 1 large banana
- 2 Tbsp collagen hydrolysate (this form of gelatin doesn't gel)
- 1 Tbsp cacao powder
- 1 Tbsp maca powder

Directions:

1. Blend and enjoy!

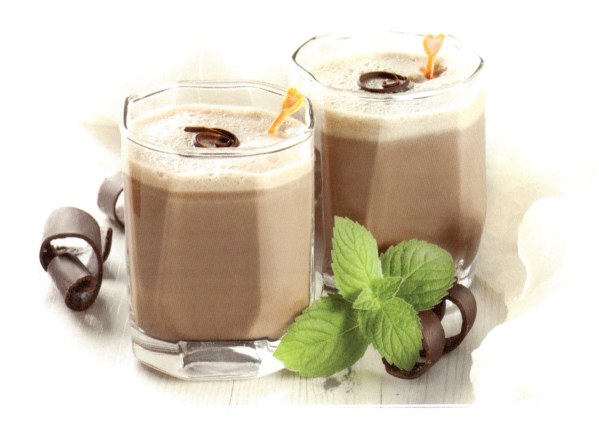

GO GREEN SMOOTHIE

Ingredients:

- ½ cup full-fat coconut milk
- ½ cup steamed (and cooled) spinach
- ½ cup ice
- 1 apple (peeled)
- 1 stalk celery
- 2 Tbsp collagen hydrolysate (this form of gelatin doesn't gel)
- 1 tsp vanilla

Directions:

1. Blend and enjoy!

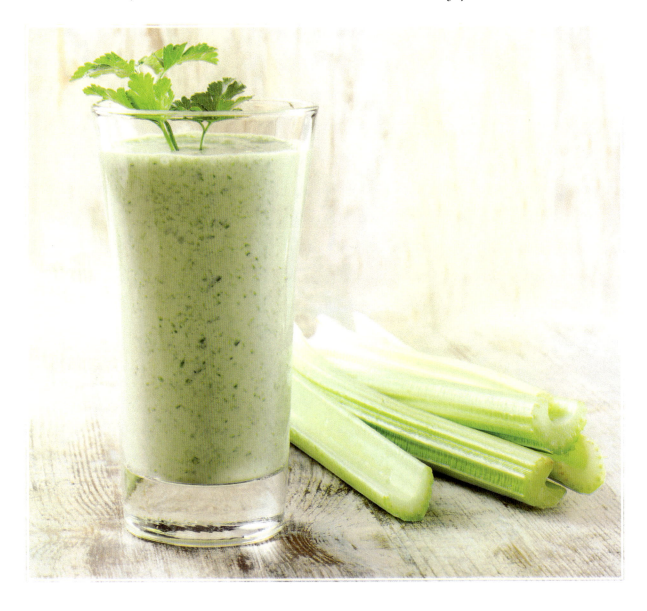

PUMPKIN BANANA SMOOTHIE

Ingredients:

- 1 cup full-fat coconut milk
- ¼ cup ice
- ¼ cup organic canned pumpkin
- 1 large banana
- 2 Tbsp collagen hydrolysate (this form of gelatin doesn't gel)
- 1 tsp pumpkin pie spice

Directions:

2. Blend and enjoy!

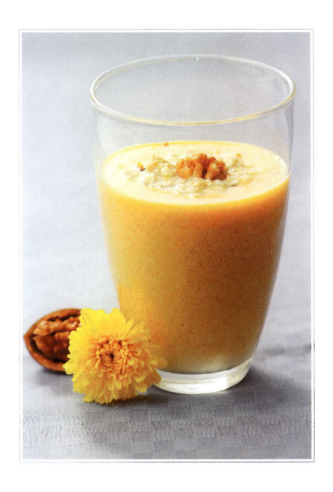

PINEAPPLE SMOOTHIE

- 1 cup full-fat coconut milk
- ⅔ cup pineapple chunks (frozen)
- ½ cup ice
- 2 Tbsp collagen hydrolysate (this form of gelatin doesn't gel)
- 1 tsp maca powder

Directions:

1. Blend and enjoy!

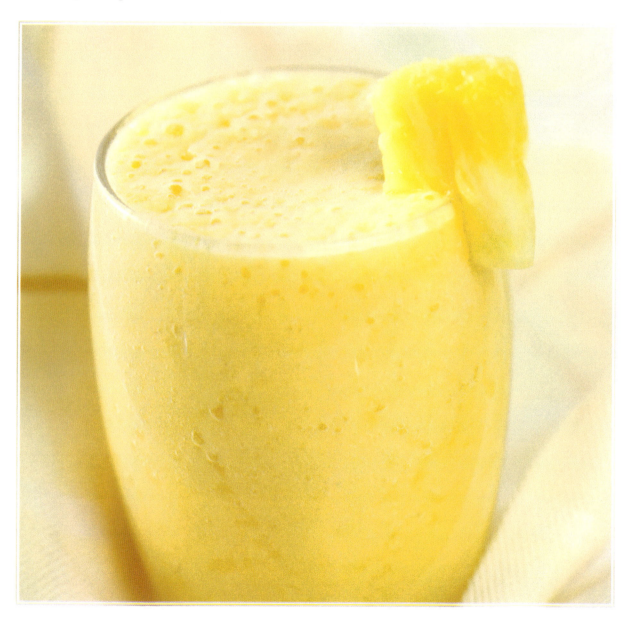

CUCUMBER AVOCADO SMOOTHIE

- 1 cup peeled sliced cucumber
- ½ banana
- ½ avocado
- ⅓ cup ice
- 2 Tbsp collagen hydrolysate (this form of gelatin doesn't gel)

Directions:

1. Blend and enjoy!

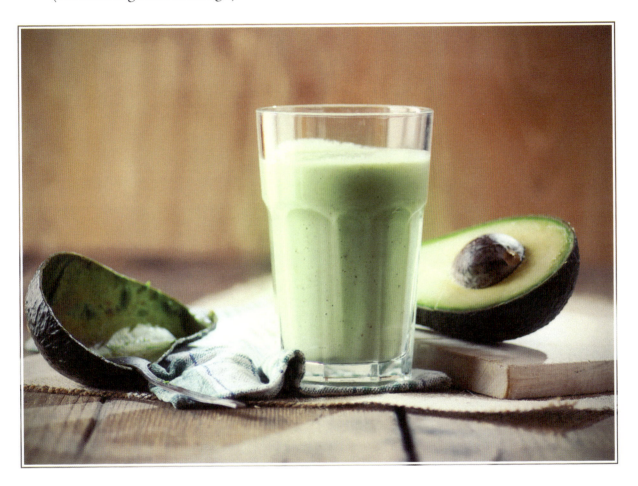

Dairy-Free Puddings and Custard

I don't know about you but sometimes this girl needs a treat. Why not make it a healthy nutrient dense treat while not making any concessions on the flavor part of the deal? These recipes are all dairy free. If you're not dairy intolerant, feel free to use milk instead. If you do, I highly recommend you use raw (unpasteurized) grass-fed milk if it's available in your area.

These would make a great dessert to serve at a dinner party. You can make them ahead of time and keep in the fridge for about a week. If you're just getting started with real foods, these are a great treat to have on hand for when your sweet tooth hits. If it helps you from diving into a bowl of chemical laden cocoa puffs, I'm all for it.

While these recipes don't contain a ton of gelatin, it is just one more idea of how you can use gelatin and how you can sneak into your diet each week.

COCONUT PUDDING

Ingredients:

- 13.5 oz (1 can) full-fat coconut milk
- ½ cup shredded coconut
- 2 Tbsp honey (preferably raw)
- 1 Tbsp gelatin
- 2 tsp vanilla extract

Directions:

1. Pour coconut milk, honey, and vanilla into a small pot and heat on med/low
2. Once heated, add gelatin
3. Use an immersion blender to help mix and dissolve gelatin
4. Turn off heat
5. Add shredded coconut and mix again with immersion blender
6. Pour into a container and let cool (a muffin tin works great for individual portions)
7. Put in the fridge for 1 hour
8. Enjoy!

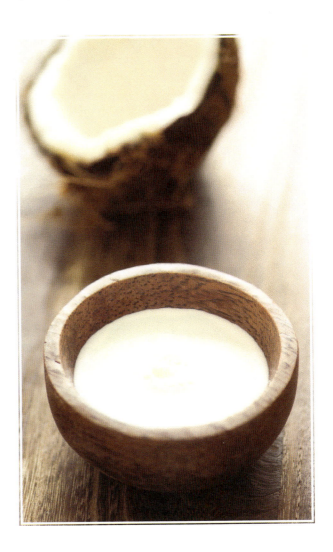

PUMPKIN PUDDING

Ingredients:

- 13.5 oz (1 can) full-fat coconut milk
- ⅓ cup puréed canned pumpkin (or make your own!)
- 1 Tbsp honey (preferably raw)
- 1 Tbsp gelatin
- 1 tsp vanilla extract
- ½ cinnamon

Directions:

1. Add all ingredients (excluding the gelatin) to small pot and warm on low/med heat
2. Use an immersion blender to blend ingredients
3. Add gelatin and mix again with the immersion blender
4. Turn off heat and pour into container to cool
5. Put in fridge for 1 hour
6. Enjoy!

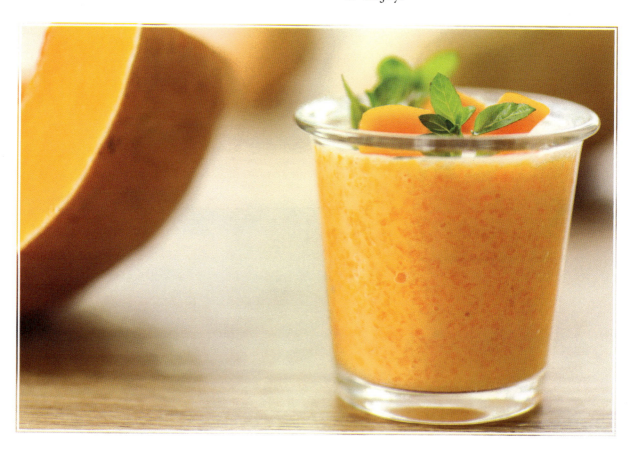

CHOCOLATE PUDDING

Ingredients:

- 13.5 oz (1 can) full-fat coconut milk
- ⅓ cup soy-free, dairy-free chocolate chips (I use Enjoy Life)
- 1 Tbsp gelatin
- 1 tsp vanilla extract
- 1 tsp honey (preferably raw)

Directions:

1. Add all ingredients (excluding the gelatin) to small pot and warm on low/med heat
2. Use the immersion blender to blend ingredients
3. Add gelatin and mix again with the immersion blender
4. Turn off heat and pour into container to cool
5. Put in fridge for 1 hour
6. Enjoy!

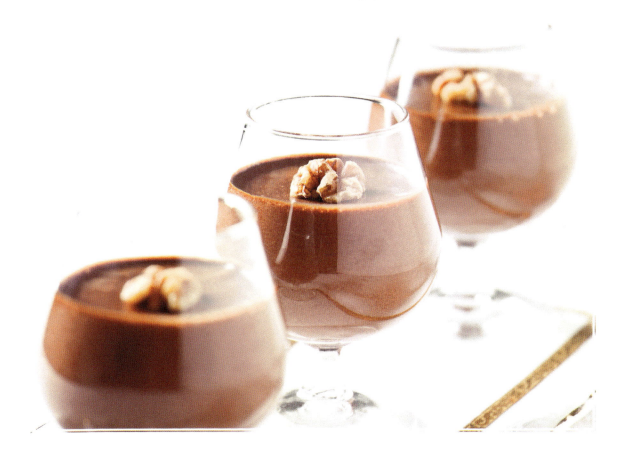

CUSTARD

Ingredients:

- 13.5 oz (1 can) full-fat coconut milk
- 4 egg yolks (preferably pastured)
- 1 Tbsp gelatin
- 1 Tbsp vanilla extract
- 1 Tbsp honey (preferably raw)

Directions:

1. Add all ingredients (excluding the gelatin) to small pot and warm on low/med heat
2. Use the immersion blender to blend ingredients
3. Add gelatin and mix again with the immersion blender
4. Turn off heat and pour into container to cool
5. Put in fridge for 1 hour
6. Enjoy!

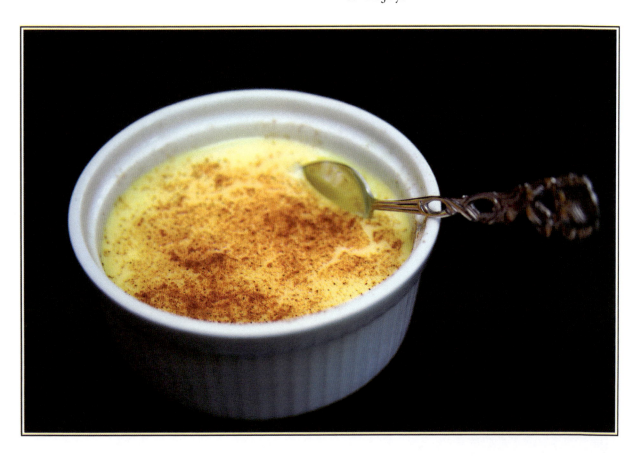

BANANA CINNAMON PUDDING

Ingredients:

- 2 large bananas, mashed
- 10 oz (about ¾ can) full-fat coconut milk
- 1 Tbsp gelatin
- 2 tsp vanilla extract
- 1 tsp honey (preferably raw)
- ½ tsp cinnamon

Directions:

1. Add all ingredients (excluding the gelatin) to small pot and warm on low/med heat
2. Use the immersion blender to blend ingredients
3. Add gelatin and mix again with the immersion blender
4. Turn off heat and pour into container to cool
5. Put in fridge for 1 hour
6. Enjoy!

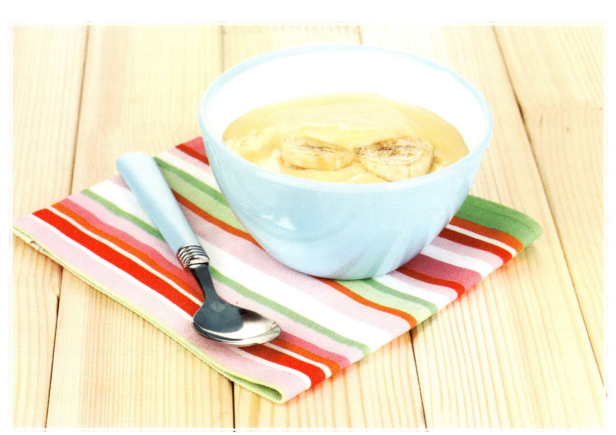

PUMPKIN CHOCOLATE MOUSSE

Ingredients:

- 13.5 oz (1 can) full-fat coconut milk
- ½ cup pumpkin purée
- ½ cup Enjoy Life chocolate chips
- 2 tsp. gelatin

Directions:

1. Heat coconut milk and chocolate chips in a pot on medium heat
2. Use an immersion blender to smooth the coconut milk/chocolate mixture
3. Add pumpkin and combine using the immersion blender
4. Turn heat off and add gelatin
5. Mix with the blender one more time
6. Pour into appropriate serving sizes
7. Place in fridge for at least 1 hour until it sets
8. Let warm to room temperature before serving
9. Enjoy!

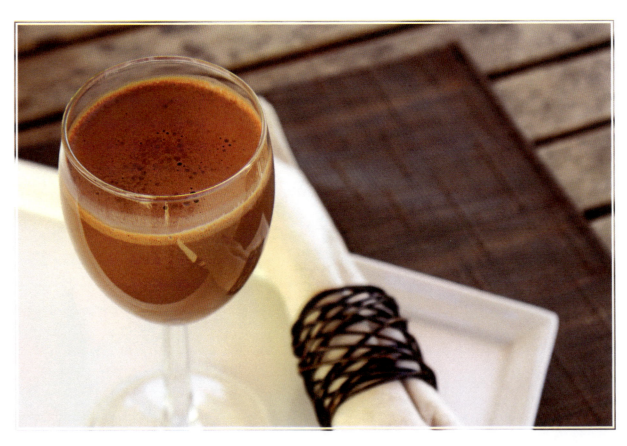

CRÈME BRÛLÉE

Ingredients:

* 13.5 oz (1 can) full-fat coconut milk
* 3 egg yolks
* ½ cup maple syrup (preferably grade B organic)
* 2 Tbsp. vanilla
* 1 tsp. gelatin

Directions:

1. Combine all ingredients (except gelatin) in a pot on medium heat
2. Use an immersion blender to mix the ingredients
3. Once the mixture is warm add the gelatin
4. Use the immersion blender to combine
5. Pour into appropriate containers and let set in the fridge for at least 1 hour
6. Let warm to room temperature
7. Enjoy!

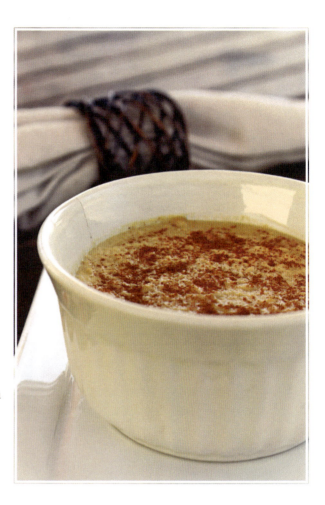

Marshmallows

CINNAMON COVERED MARSHMALLOWS (WITH CHOCOLATE DIPPED OPTION)

Ingredients:

* 3 Tbsp gelatin (the red can)
* 1 cup of filtered water divided into ½ cups
* ½ cup honey (preferably raw)
* ½ cup maple syrup (grade B organic)
* 2 tsp. vanilla
* 2 tsp. arrowroot powder
* 2 tsp. cinnamon
* ¼ tsp sea salt
* Parchment paper

Directions:

1. Line an 8x8 baking dish with parchment paper and grease with a small amount of coconut oil
2. Sprinkle the cinnamon/arrowroot powder mix on the parchment paper and spread evenly
3. Warm ½ cup of water on low heat and combine with gelatin and mix well (I use an immersion blender for this)
4. Pour the remaining ½ cup of water in small pot and combine with honey, maple syrup and salt
5. Heat on medium-high for approximately 10 minutes on your large burner
6. Once finished, immediately but SLOWLY combine the gelatin and honey mixture into a bowl with mixer on highest setting
7. Mix on high until color lightens and the mixture becomes light and fluffy (this may take up to 10 minutes)
8. Pour mixture into prepared 8x8 baking dish and let cool in the fridge for 1 to 4 hours depending on how firm you want the marshmallows (less time = less firm)

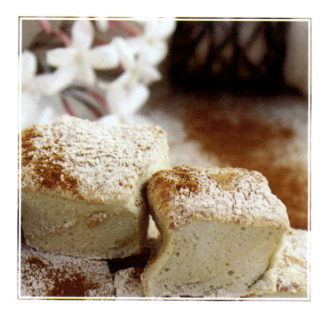

CHOCOLATE DIP

Ingredients:

- ⅓ cup soy-free, dairy-free chocolate chips (I use Enjoy Life)
- ¼ cup coconut oil

Directions:

1. Combine in a small sauce pan on med/low heat and then let cool
2. Dip firm marshmallows into chocolate, sprinkle some shredded coconut on top and place in the fridge for 30 minutes
3. Enjoy!

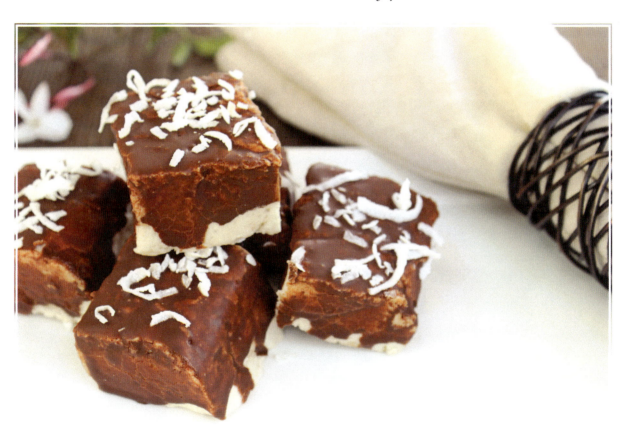

References

1. Di Lullo, GA, SM Sweeney, J Korkko, L Ala-Kokko, and JD San Antonio. "Mapping the ligand-binding sites and disease-associated mutations on the most abundant protein in the human, type I collagen." *The Journal of Biological Chemistry* 277:6 (8 Feb 2002): 4223-31. Web.

2. Houck, JC, VK Sharma, YM Patel, and JA Gladner. "Induction of collagenolytic and proteolytic activities by anti-inflammatory drugs in the skin and fibroblast." *Biochemical Pharmacology* 17:10 (Oct 1968): 2081-90. Web.

3. Daniel, Kaayla T. "Why Broth is Beautiful: Essential Roles for Proline, Glycine and Gelatin." *Weston A. Price Foundation*, 18 June 2003. Web. 10 March 2014.

4. Brinson, Linda C. "What Exactly is Jell-O Made From?" *How Stuff Works*. TLC, n.d. Web. 10 March 2014.

5. Sikorski, Zdzislaw E. *Chemical and Functional Properties of Food Proteins*. Boca Raton: CRC Press.

6. Pete, Ray. "Gelatin, stress, longevity." *Ray Peat*, 2009. Web. 10 March 2014.

7. "How to Select Collagen Supplements." *Dr. Wellness*, n.d. Web. 10 March 2014.

8. Micleu, Cindy. "Bone Broth for Health Building: Nourishing the Liver and Kidneys." *Jade Institute*, n.d. Web. 10 March 2014.

9. Mercola, Joseph. "Why Grassfed Animal Products Are Better For You." *Mercola*, n.d. Web. 10 march 2014.

10. Sisson, Mark. "Cooking with Bones." *Mark's Daily Apple*, 15 April 2010. Web. 10 March 2014.

11. Vien, Anya. "Unbelievable Health Benefits of Bone Marrow that You Should Know." *LA Healthy Living*, 28 June 2013. Web. 10 March 2014.

12. Sisson, Mark. "Bone Marrow: Delicious, Nutritious and Underappreciated." *Mark's Daily Apple*, 7 April 2010. Web. 10 March 2014.

13. Schoenfeld, Laura. "The Role of Nutrition in Collagen Production." *Ancestralize Me*, 22 April 2012. Web. 10 March 2014.

14. Katie — Wellness Mama. "Why I've Been Drinking Green Jello (Well, Almost)." *Wellness Mama*, n.d. Web. 10 March 2014.

15. Petchey, Fiona. "Bone." *C14 Dating*, n.d. Web. 10 March 2014.

16. "What is Bone?" *National Institute of Arthritis and Musculoskeletal and Skin Diseases*. National Institute of Health, January 2012. Web. 10 March 2014.

17. "Bone Fracture Healing Explained." *Physioroom*, Web. 10 March 2014.
18. Kresser, Chris. "Vitamin K2: The Missing Nutrient." *Chris Kresser*, n.d. Web. 10 March 2014.
19. Brody, Jane E. "Thinking Twice About Calcium Supplements." *The New York Times*, 8 April 2013. Web. 10 March 2014.
20. Rettner, Raechel. "Vitamin D & Calcium May Not Prevent Postmenopausal Fractures." *Live Science*, 25 February 2013. Web. 10 March 2014.
21. Wolfe, Liz. "Calcium Without Diary." *Liz Wolfe, NTP*, n.d. Web. 10 March 2014.
22. US Surgeon General. *Bone Health and Osteoporosis: A Report of the Surgeon General*. Rockville (MD): Office of the Surgeon General (US), 2004.
23. "Epidemiology." *International Osteoporosis Foundation*, n.d. Web. 10 March 2014.
24. "What is Osteoporosis?" *International Osteoporosis Foundation*, n.d. Web. 10 March 2014.
25. *Health in Your Hands: Your Plan for Natural Scoliosis Prevention and Treatment*. Dir. Kevin Lau. Perf. Darren Stephen Lim and Jason Chee. Health In Your Hands, 2011. DVD.
26. "Scoliosis: Exercise, Diet and Yoga Alternative Treatments." Sandy Simmon's Connective Tissue Disorder Site. *Pine Canyon Media*, n.d. Web. 10 March 2014.
27. Sponseller. Paul. "What is Scoliosis?" *Osteogenesis Imperfecta Foundation*, 2005. Web. 10 March 2014.
28. Simon, Harvey. "Scoliosis." *University of Maryland Medical Center*, 26 May 2012. Web. 10 March 2014.
29. Topiwala, Sheshzad "Osteomalacia." Medline Plus. *National Institute of Health,* 19 July 2012. Web. 10 March 2014.
30. "The Return of Rickets." Daily Mail. *Associated Newspapers LTD,* n.d. Web. 10 March 2014.
31. "Introduction to Bone Biology: All About Our Bones." *International Osteoporosis Foundation,* n.d. Web. 10 March 2014.
32. Oesser, S, M Adam, W Babel, and J Seifert. "Oral administration of ^{14}C labelled gelatine hydrolysate leads to an accumulation of radioactivity in cartilage of mice (C57/BL)". *Journal of Nutrition* 129:10 (Oct 1999). Web.
33. Iwai, K, T Haseqawa, Y Taquchi, F Morimatsu, K Sato, Y Nakamura, A Hiqashi, Y Kido, Y Nakabo, and K Ohtsuki. "Identification of food-derived collagen peptides in human blood after oral ingestion of gelatin hydrolysates." *Journal of Agriculture and Food Chemistry* 53:16 (Aug 2005) 6531-6. Web.
34. "Hydrolyzed Collagen." *The Doctor Within,* n.d. Web. 10 March 2014.

35. Benfit, Emily. "Guide to Choosing Gelatin Powder: Which Kind Should You Buy?" *Butter Believer*, 30 May 2013. Web. 10 March 2014.

36. Takeda, Satoko, Jong-Hoon Park, Eriko Kawashima, Ikuko Ezawa, and Naomi Omi. Hydrolyzed collagen intake increases bone mass of growing rats trained with running exercise" *Journal of the International Society of Sports Nutrition* 10:35 (2013). Web.

37. Pluvinet, Renaud, Taffin, and Audrey. "Hydrolyzed collagen: a versatile protein for joint and bone health, nutrition and beauty." *Nutraceutical Business and Technology* (Nov 2008). Web.

38. Brown, Susan E. "How to Speed Fracture Healing." Better Bones. *Center for Better Bones,* n.d. Web. 10 March 2014.

39. "Bone Fracture Healing Explained: Hard Callus Formation." *Physioroom*, n.d. Web. 10 March 2014.

40. "The Science Behind Bone Stimulation." Exogen. *Bioventus LLC,* n.d. Web. 10 March 2014.

41. Sarl, Nealth. "Biological Bone Markers and Hydrolyzed Collagen Supplement in Menopausal Healthy Women." Clinicaltrials.gov, February 2011. Web. 10 March 2014.

42. Lerche Davis, Jeanie. "Joint Pain Not Inevitable With Age." *Web MD,* 2003. Web. 10 March 2014.

43. "Joint Pain."*Web MD,* 2012. Web. 10 March 2014.

44. "Bone Broth: Health Benefits." *Primally Inspired,* n.d. Web. 10 March 2014.

45. *Arthritis Foundation.* Web. 10 March 2014. <www.arthritis.org>

46. Zhong, Z, MD Wheeler, X Li, M Froh, P Schemmer, M Yin, H Bunzendaul, B Bradford, and JJ Lemasters. "L-Glycine: a novel antiinflammatory, immunomodulatory, and cytoprotective agent." *Current Opinion in Clinical Nutrition and Metabolic Care* 6:2 (March 2003). Web.

47. "Questions and Answers: NIH Glucosamine/Chondroitin Arthritis Intervention Trial Primary Study." National Center for Complementary and Alternative Medicine. *National Institute of Health,* October 2008. Web. 10 March 2014.

48. "Proline." *OrthoMolecular,* n.d. Web. 10 March 2014.

49. Sandberg, Larry. "What is the Basic Difference between Collagen and Elastin in Skin Care?" PHD Peptides. *Discover the Science,* 11 November 2011. Web. 10 March 2014.

50. "Biotin and Probiotics." *Vitamin Information Center.* Web. <www.vic-japan.gr.jp/vic/106/106e.pdf>

51. Mercola, Joseph. "How Your Gut Flora Influences Your Health." *Mercola,* 27 June 2012. Web. 10 March 2014.

52. Sanfilippo, Diane. "Is Your Gut Lucky?" *Balanced Bites*, July 2010. Web. 10 march 2014.

53. Jaminet, Paul. "Wheat Is A Cause of Many Diseases, I: Leaky Gut." *Perfect Health Diet*, 26 October 2010. Web. 10 March 2014.

54. Croxton, Sean. "Top 5 Reasons Why Bone Broth is The Bomb." *Underground Wellness*, 17 October 2012. Web. 10 March 2014.

55. Wang, W, S Uzzau, SE Goldblum, and A Fasano. "Human zonulin, a potential modulator of intestinal tight junctions." *Journal of Cell Science* 113:24 (Dec 2000). Web.

56. "Are GMOs Increasing the Incidence of Gluten Sensitivities?" *Nourishing Meals*, 11 October 2012. Web. 10 March 2014.

57. Reasoner, Jordan. "Leaky Gut Syndrome In Plain English — And How To Fix It." *SCD Lifestyle,* March 2010. Web. 10 March 2014.

58. Hawser. Stephen P and Khalid Islam. "Binding of Candida albicans to Immobilized Amino Acids and Bovine Serum Albumin." *Infection and Immunity* 66:1 (Jan 1998). Web.

59. Simon, Martin. "Intestinal Permeability." *BioMed Newsletter* (11 May 1995). *Anapsid.org*. Web. 10 March 2014.

60. Weil, Andrew. "What Is Leaky Gut?" *Dr. Weil*, 12 December 2005. Web. 10 March 2014.

61. Kresser, Chris. "9 Steps to Perfect Health — #5: Heal Your Gut." *Chris Kesser*, Web. 10 March 2014.

62. Simon, Martin. "Intestinal Permeability." *BioMed Newsletter* (11 May 1995). *Anapsid.org*. Web. 10 March 2014.

63. Axe, Josh. "4 Steps to Heal Leaky Gut and Autoimmune Disease." *Draxe*, n.d. Web. 10 March 2014.

64. "What is the Difference Between a Food Allergy, Food Intolerance and Food Sensitivity?" *Institute of Food Technologists,* n.d. Web. 10 March 2014.

65. Kresser, Chris. "50 Shades of Gluten Intolerance." *Chris Kresser*, n.d. Web. 10 March 2014.

66. Morris, Megan. "Leaky Gut." *The Root Of Health*, 2011. Web. 10 March 2014.

67. Ballantyne, Sarah. *The Paleo Approach: Reverse Autoimmune Disease and Heal Your Body.* Victory Belt Publishing, 2014. eBook.

68. "IgG ELISA Delayed Food Allergy Testing." *Dr Braly Allergy Relief*, n.d. Web. 10 March 2014.

69. Ferguson, Kellie. "Food Sensitivity Testing — Let's Talk About Your Options!" *The Paleo Mom*, 6 September 2012. Web. 10 March 2014.

70. Robbins, Albert. "Food Allergy and IgA deficiency." *Foods Matter*, August 2010. Web. 10 March 2014.

71. "Food Reactions." *Rocky Mountain Analytical*, n.d. Web. 10 March 2014.

72. Allbritton, Jen. "Soup-Stenance." *Weston A. Price Foundation*, 27 March 2012. Web. 10 March 2014.

73. Bardelli, Carol. "Nutrition 101: What is Gluconeogenesis?" *Examiner*, 21 August 2009. Web. 10 March 2014.

74. "Glycine." ImageryNet. *The Gersten Institute*, n.d. Web. 10 March 2014.

75. Serwach, Joe. "Bitter truth: Stress Drives Sweet Craving." The University Record. *The University of Michigan*, 17 April 2006. Web. 10 March 2014.

76. Veldhorst, et al. "A breakfast with alpha-lactalbumin, gelatin, or gelatin + TRP lowers energy intake at lunch compared with a breakfast with casein, soy, whey, or whey-GMP." *Clinical Nutrition* 28:2 (April 2009). Web.

77. "Diet Myth News Flash: Eating Less Does Not Cause Fat Loss." *Ben Green Field Fitness*, n.d. Web. 10 March 2014.

78. Boston, Gabriella. "Basal Metabolic Rate Changes As You Age." *Washington Post*, 6 March 2013. Web. 10 March 2014.

79. Wells, Wendy. "The Brain Game, Balancing Neurotransmitters and Hormones." *Heart Spring*, n.d. Web. 10 March 2014.

80. Sahelian, Ray. "Cortisol Hormone High Level and Side Effects, How to Reduce, Risks and Danger." *Ray Sahelian*, n.d. Web. 10 March 2014.

81. "What is Adrenal Fatigue?" *Adrenal Fatigue*, n.d. Web. 10 March 2014.

82. "Being Hangry: The Neuroscience behind Hunger and a Sour Mood." *Health Medicine Network*, n.d. Web. 10 March 2014.

83. Nordqvist, Christian. "What is Serotonin? What does Serotonin Do?" *Medical News Today*, 3 November 2013. Web. 10 March 2014.

84. Wolfe, Liz. *Skintervention Guide: Purely Paleo Skincare*. 2013. eBook.

85. Kresser, Chris. "RHR: Naturally Get Rid Of Acne By Fixing Your Gut." *Chris Kresser*, n.d. Web. 10 March 2014.

86. Garnas, Eirik. "Acne Originates in the Gut." *Organic Fitness*, 9 June 2012. Web. 10 March 2014.

87. "Probiotics Send Signals From Your Gut to Your Skin." *Mercola*, 11 November 2011. Web. 10 March 2014.

88. Heino, Katja. "Gelatin: Do You Know this Superfood?" *Savory Lotus*, 22 May 2013. Web. 10 March 2014.

89. "Hormonal Acne: Where It's Coming From, and What to Do about It." *Paleo For Women*, n.d. Web. 10 March 2014.

90. Bartlett, Emily. *The Eczema Cure: Heal from the Inside Out with Real Food.* eBook.

91. Barrymore, John. "Collagen Injections Overview." How Stuff Works. *TLC,* n.d. Web. 10 March 2014.

92. Rogers, Amber. "Cellulite: It's Time We All Just Get the Hell Over It." *Go Kaleo.* 6 March 2013. Web. 10 March 2014.

93. "Everything You Need To Know About Why You Get Cellulite And How To Get Rid Of Cellulite." *Ben Green Field Fitness*, 8 May 2012. Web. 10 March 2014.

94. Turner, Natasha. "Four Ways to Combat Cellulite." *Huffington Post*, 20 December 2012. Web. 10 March 2014.

95. "Hair Growth—Hair Construction." *Hair Finder*, n.d. Web. 10 March 2014.

96. "Production of the Hair by the Follicle." *Centre Clauderer*, n.d. Web. 10 March 2014.

97. "What is hair made of?" *Grow Hair Guru*, n.d. Web. 10 March 2014.

98. Meneses, Monique. "Collagen: An Important Ingredient for Youthful Hair." *New Beauty*, 17 April 2012. Web. 10 March 2013.

99. "Keratin and Collagen." *Wiley*, n.d. Web. 10 March 2014.

100. Smith, Tara. "Bad Hair Day? Blame Your Shampoo." *My Pure Radiance,* 19 July 2013. Web. 10 March 2014.

101. "Foods to Eat for Healthy Teeth and Nails." *Delicious Magazine*, n.d. Web. 10 March 2014.

102. Melina, Remy. "Why Are Teeth Not Considered Bones?" *Live Science*, 18 March 2011. Web. 10 March 2014.

103. "Dental Pulp." *University of Kentucky*, n.d. Web. 10 March 2014.

104. Nagel, Ramiel. *Cure Tooth Decay: Heal and Prevent Cavities with Nutrition*. CreateSpace Independent Publishing Platform, 2010. eBook.

105. Fallon Morell, Sally. "Ancient Dietary Wisdom for Tomorrow's Children." *Weston A. Price Foundation*, 1 January 2000. Web. 10 March 2014.

106. Katie—The Paleo Mama. "How I'm Healing My Cavities Without Dentistry." *The Paleo Mama*, 26 November 2013. Web. 10 March 2014.

107. Boskey, Adele L. "Mineralization of Bones and Teeth." *Elements* V.3 (December 2007): 387-393. Web.

108. "How Bone Broths Support Your Adrenals, Bones and Teeth." *Nourished Kitchen*, 14 June 2012. Web. 10 March 2010.

109. "Bone Broth Battle: Chicken Vs. Beef…FIGHT!" *Paleohacks*, 28 November 2011. Web. 10 March 2010.

110. Sisson Mark. "Beef Bone Broth vs. Chicken." *Mark's Daily Apple*, 23 November 2011. Web. 10 March 2010.

111. Bauman, Diana. "The Miracles of Broth." *My Humble Kitchen*, 28 October 2009. Web. 10 March 2014.

112. Fallon, Sally and Mary Enig. *Nourishing Traditions: The Cookbook that Challenges Politically Correct Nutrition and the Diet Dictocrats.* Newtrends Publishing, 2003.

113. "What is the Ideal Fish for Making FISH bone broth?" *Paleohacks*, 12 December 2012. Web. 10 March 2014.

114. Alfaro, Danilo. "Fish Stock Recipe." Culinary Arts. *About.com*, n.d. Web. 10 March 2014.

115. Matheson, Lauren. "How to Make Bone Broth with Serious Gel." *Kitchen Stewardship*. 15 November 2011. Web. 10 March 2014.

116. Sarah — The Health Home Economist. "5 Reasons Why Your Stock Won't Gel." The Healthy Home Economist. *Austus Foods*, 31 March 2012. Web. 10 March 2014.